Meeting the Challenges of Elder Care

Japan and Norway

Meeting the Challenges of Elder Care

Japan and Norway

edited by

Yayoi Saito,

Reiko Abe Auestad

and

Kari Wærness

Kyoto University Press

TRANS PACIFIC PRESS

First published in 2010 jointly by:

Kyoto University Press
Kyodai Kaikan
15-9 Yoshida Kawara-cho
Sakyo-ku, Kyoto 606-8305, Japan
Telephone: +81-75-761-6182
Fax: +81-75-761-6190
Email: sales@kyoto-up.or.jp
Web: http://www.kyoto-up.or.jp

Trans Pacific Press
PO Box 164, Balwyn North, Melbourne
Victoria 3104, Australia
Telephone: +61 3 9859 1112
Fax: +61 3 9859 4110
Email: tpp.mail@gmail.com
Web: http://www.transpacificpress.com

Distributors

Australia and New Zealand
DA Information Services/Central Book Services
648 Whitehorse Road
Mitcham, Victoria 3132
Australia
Telephone: +61(0)3-9210-7777
Fax: + 61(0)3-9210-7788
Email: books@dadirect.com
Web: www.dadirect.com

USA and Canada
International Specialized Book Services
(ISBS)
920 NE 58th Avenue, Suite 300
Portland, Oregon 97213-3786
USA
Telephone: (800) 944-6190
Fax: (503) 280-8832
Email: orders@isbs.com
Web: http://www.isbs.com

Asia and the Pacific
Kinokuniya Company Ltd.

Head office:
38-1 Sakuragaoka 5-chome
Setagaya-ku, Tokyo 156-8691
Japan
Telephone: +81(0)3-3439-0161
Fax: +81(0)3-3439-0839
Email: bkimp@kinokuniya.co.jp
Web: www.kinokuniya.co.jp

Asia-Pacific office:
Kinokuniya Book Stores of Singapore Pte., Ltd.
391B Orchard Road #13-06/07/08
Ngee Ann City Tower B
Singapore 238874
Telephone: +65 6276 5558
Fax: +65 6276 5570
Email: SSO@kinokuniya.co.jp

ISBN 978–1–920901–95–0

Contents

Figures

Tables

List of Contributors

Kari Wærness (born 1939) has been Professor of Sociology at the University of Bergen since 1987. She obtained Candidata Magisterii of Science at the University of Bergen in 1963 and Honorary Doctor at the University of Uppsala in 2004. Her research has covered the areas of social policy and family sociology, with particular emphasis on the work on women, and the relation between unpaid care in families and the formally organized health and social services. She is currently engaged in a research project, 'Globalization and Changes in the Cultures of Survival and Care,' which is connected to the Institute of African Studies, University of Ghana, Legon.

Karen Christensen (born 1959) is Associate Professor at the Department of Sociology, University of Bergen. With her thesis 'Care and Work: A Sociological Study about Changes in Norwegian Home Based Care Services,' she became PhD of Sociology in 1997 at the University of Bergen. She has since researched and published in areas such as the modernization of social care services, care policy practices, and care and disability. Among several articles, she has co-authored a status report on Norwegian care services. She has also been an editor of *the Norwegian Journal of Sociology*. Her central interests are social care and services, social policy, the challenges of the welfare state, and qualitative methodology.

Yayoi Saito (born 1964) is Associate Professor in social welfare studies in the Graduate School of Human Sciences, Osaka University. She completed a Master's Degree of Public Administration at the Department of Political Science, University of Lund, in 1993. She has been a guest researcher at the University of Lund (2002), the University of Växjö (2002), and the University of Oslo (2008). She has published books and articles on elderly care in Sweden. She has also researched elderly care in Japan and works as a committee member of the Long-Term Care Insurance Management Committee in several municipalities. Her central interests are international comparative studies of elderly care.

Reiko Abe Auestad (born 1956) is Professor at the Department of Culture Studies and Oriental Languages, University of Oslo. She has a Master's Degree (University of Wisconsin) and a PhD (University of Oslo) in Japanese literature, and has published books and articles on Japanese authors such as

Sōseki Natsume, Ogai Mori, Osamu Dazai, and Haruki Murakami. She has also written about Henrik Ibsen and about Norwegian society in general. Her chapter on the Japanese Long-Term Care Insurance System in the present volume will also appear in *Japan Forum*, a journal of the British Association for Japanese Studies.

Unni Edvardsen (born 1965) is Performance Auditor at Salten Kommunerevisjon, an inter-municipal local government entity. She wrote her master's thesis within political science at the University of Bergen, focusing on Japanese politics. She was a Monbusho (Ministry of Education, Culture, Sports, Sciences, and Technology in Japan) scholar at Meiji University, 1994–1995. She has worked both within academia and as a public servant. She was a research fellow for four years at the Department of Sociology and Political Science at the Norwegian University of Science and Technology (2002–2006). Her central interests are elderly care studies and policy implementation analysis within social care.

Norio Okazawa (born 1944) has been Professor at the Graduate School of Social Sciences, Waseda University, since 1981. He holds a PhD in International Studies, Waseda University, and his areas of specialty include political science and the comparative study of political system. A doyen of Scandinavian studies in Japan, he has published numerous books on the political systems and societies in Nordic countries. For his many years of contribution in promoting the study of Sweden in Japan, he was awarded the Order of the Pole Star 'Kommendör av Kungl. Nordstjärneorden' from H.M. King of Sweden in 1992. He also launched several book projects on Norway in Japan and was awarded the Royal Norwegian Order of Merit 'Kommendør av Den Kongelige Norske Fortjenstorden' from HM King of Norway in 2008. His knowledge as an expert on Scandinavia is sought after, and he works as a member of several national and local government committees.

Translator (Chapter 3 and 6)

Beverley Anne Yamamoto is Associate Professor in the Graduate School of Human Sciences, Osaka University. She was awarded a PhD in East Asian Studies from the University of Sheffield, United Kingdom, in 1999 for her research on youth sexual behavior and gender in Japan. While continuing to conduct research on youth sexuality, current projects include the experiences of children of mixed heritage growing up in Japan and the life stories of women leading unconventional lives in Japan. Major translations include Chizuko Ueno's highly acclaimed *Nationalism and Gender* (2004), Part 2 (Women and Health) of *Women, Gender and Human Rights: A Global Perspective* edited by Marjorie Agosin (2007), and, with Jennifer Igawa, *Media Literacy Education for Japanese Pre-School and Elementary School Children* by Mami Komaya (forthcoming, Spring 2010).

Introduction

As with most academic collaborations, there is a history to this book. Alongside Norio Okazawa (Waseda University), we, Reiko Abe Auestad (University of Oslo) and Yayoi Saito (Osaka University), participated in a Japanese book project about Norway, which resulted in an introductory three-volume publication from Waseda University Press in 2005 on Norwegian society, economics, and politics. This project was originally planned as part of the celebration of the anniversary of the establishing of diplomatic relations between the two countries. The project gave the three of us an opportunity to consider in greater depth not only the many obvious differences between the two countries, but also their broader meaning given that Japan and Norway, as industrialized nations in the late modern phase, would face many similar challenges in the future. We set out with the expectation that this line of enquiry would shed greater light on the current and future situations in both countries, as it did.

From the Japanese perspective, the impact of a rapidly ageing population combined with an alarmingly low birthrate had already emerged as a pressing problem, and it was apparent that there was an urgent need to discuss the various forms of social welfare needed to address it. Likewise, Norway was also experiencing the same problems, albeit to a more moderate degree. A question has been raised in the national media over whether – given the worsening situation – Norway really deserved to be called a welfare state in the area of the elderly care.

The concrete idea for a comparative project on the elderly care in Norway and Japan came from Auestad, who has spent most of her adult life in Norway but has had the responsibility of caring for ageing parents living in Tokyo. Kindly hosted by Okazawa, Auestad spent a few months as guest researcher at Waseda University in 2004 and 2005, which gave her an opportunity to begin her research on the elderly care in Japan. Part of the stay was financed by the Scandinavia-Japan Sasakawa Foundation. Looking for Norwegian research partners, Auestad came across Kari Wærness's paper 'On the Rationality of Caring' which is reproduced in the first chapter of the present anthology (the content of the essay will be summarized later). Inspired by Wærness's ideas, Auestad contacted her to ask whether she would be interested in collaboration.

One of the features of this anthology is that, while all the papers share the common objective of addressing the problem of elderly care in Japan and Norway, each approaches the issue from a unique perspective based on discipline, research focus, and linguistic and cultural background. For example, Auestad, is a specialist in Japanese literature and does not have an academic background in sociology or social welfare. None of the contributors is a native speaker of English. Some have written their chapters directly in English, while others have had them translated. As a result there are more than a few stylistic differences. Anchored in a different tradition of essay writing, the definition of an academic article in Japan differs somewhat from that found in Norway or elsewhere. Conventions concerning publication are also a little different. In this respect, we would particularly like to acknowledge the contribution of Dr Beverley Anne Yamamoto (Associate Professor, Osaka University) for not only translating two of the chapters, but also for her editing advice. In addition, as a gender studies specialist raised in Britain but with many years of experience living in Japan, she was able to offer input on the gender dimensions of the elderly care issue.

It is our hope that these variations of style, perspective and, at times, even interpretation, will be considered our strength rather than a weakness in that this book represents not only the outcome but also the positive possibilities of cooperation across the linguistic, cultural, and disciplinary boundaries in the increasingly globalized world in which we all now live.

Our shared experiences of research exchange

This book was the result of active research collaboration between the various authors. We would like to briefly outline the various research and study meetings that we conducted so that our readers can gain some insight into the collaborative process that led to this volume.

Tokyo, December 2006

With the financial support of Grants-in-Aid for Scientific Research (*Kakenhi*) in 2005–2007 by the Japan Society for the Promotion of Science (JSPS), Saito organized a workshop at Waseda University in December 2005 (kindly hosted by Okazawa, a pioneer of Scandinavian Studies in Japan), inviting Kari Wærness (University of Bergen), Karen Christensen (University of Bergen), and Unni Edvardsen (Norwegian University of Science and Technology) from Norway. Junichi Hisatsuka, professor of Waseda University, and Auestad were also among the participation. In addition to the workshop, Saito arranged some study visits in Tokyo. After a short lecture on the Long-Term Care Insurance System at the city office of the Nishi-Tokyo Municipality, we had the opportunity to discuss the challenges of the new system with those working on the frontline. Furthermore, we visited a not-for-profit (NPO) care provider called *Nenrin* (literally, *annual growth ring* in English). Ms Atsuko Yasuoka, the chief director of *Nenrin,* helped to pioneer twenty-four-hour home help services in Japan in the 1990s. We were able to observe the work of the ordinary home helper visiting the home of an elderly person and also to speak with family carers and care workers in Nishi-Tokyo. *Rengo*, the Japanese Trade Union Confederation, also provided us with useful information about working condition of female workers in Japan.

Bergen, August 2007

Saito visited the Norwegian scholars at the University of Bergen the following summer with the help of a JSPS grant. Wærness and Christensen kindly arranged a research seminar at the Department of Sociology, University of Bergen. Saito gave a presentation entitled 'Recent Developments in Japanese Welfare States and the Japanese Elderly Care.' This provided an opportunity to further discuss our research and exchange information. Saito received useful feedback from the Norwegian scholars. In addition, Christensen kindly arranged some study visits focusing on elderly care in Bergen. It was the first opportunity for Saito to observe the work of home helpers in Norway. She interviewed Ms Gunvor Møller, former director of nursing and care section in Fana district in the Municipality of Bergen, and some other persons working in elderly care.

Trondheim, September 2007

The Japan Program at the Norwegian University of Science and Technology holds a research seminar almost every year in Trondheim. In 2007 the organizers planned a seminar entitled 'Elder Care in Japan and Norway' to discuss elderly care in each country. The seminar was financially supported by the Japan Foundation. Dr Paul Midford (Professor, Norwegian University of Science and Technology) was program director and Edvardsen, research fellow, contributed to the organizing of the program. Edvardsen gave a paper entitled 'Assessments and the Allocation of Eldercare in Japan and Norway.' Saito also gave a paper, 'Care Providers in the Long-Term Care Insurance System in Japan – The potential of and challenges faced by social enterprises.' Dr John Creighton Campbell (Professor, University of Michigan), an expert in the comparative study of elderly care systems, was present at the seminar and gave the audience valuable feedback, as did many of the participants.

Oslo, August – September 2008

Saito spent two months as a guest researcher at the University of Oslo in 2008 with a scholarship from The Research Council of Norway. During the period, Auestad and Saito visited elderly care homes in Oslo and interviewed directors and workers. Saito also visited home help providers in Oslo. It was during this period that we started to discuss and plan in earnest this book. In connection with this, we visited Wærness and Christensen in Bergen to receive their advice.

This book involved a lot of long-distance travel and communication. As a result, we were able to experience and gain a deeper knowledge of elderly care in each country. We hope to further build our research collaboration in the future.

The welfare systems in Norway and Japan and the outline of the book

The welfare system in Norway is categorized as a variant of the social democratic, Nordic welfare-state model, and shares many characteristics with that of Sweden, Denmark, Finland, and Iceland. The public sector plays a bigger role in all of the Nordic countries as a provider of social welfare than in most other industrialized nations, even though there are differences among them. According to Olof Petersson, Sweden is the prototype with the most prominent 'Nordic' characteristics. In contrast, the public sector in Iceland is relatively small, and Denmark relies on a relatively large private sector to provide welfare services and pensions. In the face of the economic crisis in the 1980s, Denmark and Sweden had to cut down on public expenditure, coping with a deficit and a rising unemployment rate in the 1990s. Norway has enjoyed revenues from oil and natural gas, and has thus been able to compensate for the difficult economic situation.

The social welfare system in Japan, on the other hand, is more difficult to categorize. Some argue that it resembles Esping-Andersen's *conservative and strongly corporatist* model typically seen in Germany, as it relies on social insurance rather than tax-financed measures. Others classify it as a variant of the *liberal, Anglo-Saxon* model, because social welfare is limited in scope and is primarily targeted at the needy, while the principle of the market economy reigns in the extent to which it caters to the needs of the middle class and the wealthy. Yet others have pointed out the affinity of the Japanese system with the Asian model, as the care of the elderly has been traditionally delegated to the responsibility of the family rather than the state.

Realizing, however, that the family-based welfare model cannot meet the demands of the rapidly ageing population, the Japanese government implemented various reforms in the 1990s and introduced the Long-Term Care Insurance System (*Kaigo hoken seido* – LTCI System) in 2000. The reforms and new insurance system aim to promote independence, choice, and a social service of high quality for individuals. The state manages the insurance system but allows the market to establish a network of welfare-related institutions that are paid for by insurance premiums, which are mandatory for all aged forty years old or over. The idea is to combine forces in the public and private sectors, creating social services of high quality by encouraging competition.

While the approaches employed over the years may be very different, Norway and Japan share similar problems in meeting the demands of an ageing society. Both Norway and Japan have been forced to come up with new strategies to meet the new demographic and economic challenges. Norway and other Nordic countries have tackled the increasing difficulty of shouldering the burden of caring in the public sector by relying more on the private sector, albeit in different ways and to different degrees. Denmark and Sweden have been more active in letting the private sector participate in competition with the public sector, and, although Norway is heading in the same direction, it has done so to a lesser extent and with caution. As already mentioned, Japan has introduced the LTCI System as its strategy, a system which relies much more heavily on the private sector. One can argue that, in a broad sense, the new insurance system is the long-awaited, official acknowledgment that the care of the elderly is no longer a private business but a societal problem, and that the management of it belongs to the public sector. In this sense, one can perhaps say that the Japanese model moved away from the Asian model after the introduction of the LTCI System.

Regardless of the type of welfare system, what matters in the end is the quality of *care*. The common concern in the chapters in this anthology is precisely how we can best enhance the quality of care within the context of the historical, cultural and institutional constraints in which the Norwegian and Japanese systems are embedded. We therefore begin our anthology by featuring the concept of *rationality of care* popularized by Norwegian sociologist Kari Wærness (Chapter 1, 'On the Rationality of Caring'). In the Nordic historical context, she problematizes the concept of scientific rationality that has dominated the discourse on public management in the modern and late modern phases, and argues for the importance of reconceptualizing rationality 'in relation to what most of us in our everyday lives perceive as the essential values in a *caring relationship*' (p. 3).

Chapter 2, 'Between Late Modern and Later Modern Elderly Care in Norway and Japan,' by Karen Christensen, traces the development of home help services in Norway by dividing the development into three phases: the traditional phase in the 1970s, characterized by the deployment of *housewives* and an experience-based knowledge of care; the modern phase, characterized by bureaucratization of services and professionalization of caregivers in the 1980s; and the late modern phase, driven by the ideology of the new public management in the 1990s.

Both Wærness and Christensen express concern that quality of care has been compromised in the name of professionalization and standardization, trends which started in the modern phase and have continued in the late modern phase, with ever more focus on effficiency. Christensen is particularly critical of the trend towards privatization and 'individualized care' in the late modern phase, and seems to see the system of neoliberal style public management as a barrier to realizing 'rationality of care'. Christensen also comments on the Japanese care of the elderly, arguing that it went from the traditional family-based model to the late modern phase as a result of the introduction of the new public management-inspired insurance system, and thus skipped the intermediate phase. Thus emerges as a controversial point in this volume.

In Chapter 3, 'Development of Home Help in Japan: A Comparison with Norway,' Yayoi Saito uses Christensen's three-phase scheme in analyzing the development of the Japanese home-help services. In contrast to Christensen, Saito argues that similar features characterizing the three phases in Norway have been present in Japan, but in a much more compressed form, since the history of the public home-help services is much shorter. She takes issue with Christensen's claim of the absence of the modern phase in Japan by arguing that the break with the traditional, family-based welfare system came with the Gold Plan in the 1990s. The Gold Plan finalized a gradual shift away from home help as poor relief to universal access, at least in principle. The Gold Plan reflected a growing consensus that families alone should not and could not be responsible for elderly care, and that they needed backup through the welfare system. She contends, therefore, that the Gold Plan, which involved the setting of targets for home helpers by municipalities, represented a break with the traditional model and the arrival of the modern phase. The fact that this phase lasted only a few years and overlapped the phases that preceded and followed it, however, makes it difficult to detect at first glance.

Saito also comments on the passing of the NPO Law (1998), which allowed for the greater participation of the civil society sector because voluntary organizations were able to register for NPO status. With the introduction of the LTCI Law in 2000 and the pluralization of elderly care provision, these groups were able to compete on the basis of a level playing field in a care service market with social welfare corporations (which in character appear to be more public than private sector institutions) and for-profit organizations. Saito argues that this marks the completion of the shift from Christensen's modernization to public management period.

In Chapter 4, 'Long-Term Care Insurance, Marketization, and Quality of Care: "Good Time Living,"' Auestad examines the quality of care in a Japanese private home on a micro-level from a comparative perspective and asks to what extent rationality of care is successfully implemented in the new LTCI System in Japan. Auestad argues that the insurance system, despite its problems, represents an important step away from the family-based welfare model, and that its focus on individualized care can in fact enhance the quality of care. Comparing the Japanese situation with the Norwegian one, where entry into care homes is much more limited, she indirectly problematizes the ideological skepticism towards the use of private forces that she detects among Norwegian scholars. Auestad's essay is, however, based on fieldwork done in 2006, and does not necessarily take into consideration the 'revision' of the insurance system in April 2006 and the recent financial crisis, both of which are said to have adversely affected the operation of the LTCI.

In Chapter 5, 'The Work Situations of Home Helpers in Japan and Norway,' Unni Edvardsen compares ways in which Japanese and Norwegian home helpers conduct their care work by analyzing the results of an interview survey and other empirical data. Using the concept of 'relational power,' which is closely connected to Wærness's rationality of caring, she examines 'different structural conditions for home helpers' work' and discusses 'their likely impacts on relational power' (p. 92–93). She concludes that while Norwegian workers seem to fare better in terms of 'contact with colleagues and salary,' they are in a much more pressed situation in terms of the number of clients they need to cover in a given time, which allows little possibility to cultivate personal connections: 'In Norway, structural power is more explicit, giving less space for relational power. In Japan, structures relating to this seem to allow a larger space for relational power (at least prior to the implementation of the LTCI revision in April 2006)' (p. 101). Edvardsen's finding are interesting in that they suggest that 'relational power' can be maintained under the LTCI System.

Chapter 6, 'Care Providers in Japan: The Potential of and Challenges for Social Enterprises' by Yayoi Saito examines the impact of the theories of the welfare mix and new public management on the nature of care providers in Japan with particular focus on the concept of 'social enterprises,' a concept developed by Victor Pestoff. It interestingly elucidates the various positive possibilities and potentials that exist in the concept of 'welfare mix' within the Japanese LTCI System. It also considers the issue of institutional sustainability for small non-governmental organization providers that have to rely mainly on the good will and volunteer spirit of largely female carers to provide their services.

To sum up, the Japanese contributors argue that the new Japanese insurance system, although inspired by new public management ideals, can foster possibilities for the positive development of 'welfare mix' by allowing care providers of diverse origin, structure, and missions to participate in the care of the elderly, while there seems to be more skepticism among the Norwegian contributors about the idea of 'welfare mix.' For them, letting private forces intervene in welfare management is perhaps a necessary evil, but it is by no means an ideal situation because, in Christensen's words, 'privatization, whether practiced in Japan or in Norway, tends in the long run to weaken the role of the employee' (p. 36). Both Wærness and Christensen have written on the basis of evidence that private outsourcing in the spirit of new public management has put pressure on the working conditions of care workers in Norway, making recruitment more difficult.

These different takes on the welfare mix model (sometimes known as *welfare pluralism*) can be explained partly as a result of the changed context in which the idea of 'welfare mix' has been interpreted and implemented in the two countries. Even though the idea of welfare mix was originally developed independently of the trend towards neoliberalism, the term has been appropriated by the proponents of *new public management*. As one Japanese critic points out, the term has impulses both towards privatization and neoliberalism on the one hand, and a renewed sense of social solidarity (with its focus on the civil sector) on the other hand, depending on how it is practiced (Tsubogo 2007: 228).

The anthology's closing section consists of epilogues by both Kari Wærness and Norio Okazawa, representing the Norwegian and Japanese appeals for the betterment of welfare from their respective perspectives. Reviewing the history of the public management of welfare in Norway, Wærness deplores the neoliberal turn in welfare policy and a 'new disciplinary order of managerialism' that has been 'imposed on the care workers' at the expense of the quality of care (p. 134–135). Being a major exponent of rationality of care, Wærness argues that it is 'high time to reform the services from the bottom up.' 'The important knowledge resources' represented by the 'experienced frontline workers,' which have been ignored in the efficiency-oriented new

public management regime, should be more actively utilized in 'the planning process' in the future (p. 134–135).
In his epilogue, 'Aiming towards Diversity Welfare in a Global Society,' Okazawa, on the other hand, argues for the need for *diversity management* in the increasingly globalized world in which lifestyle and work-style are diversifying. *Diversity management* is a strategy to promote the positive acknowledgment of diversity in society – diversity in terms of gender, race, age, disability, religion, and sexual orientation, factors that are known to impact on the fair treatment of people. With its focus on homogeneity and unity, Japanese society has not been known for promoting diversity in the past, a fact that Okazawa seems to take as the point of departure for his vision for the future. As he seems to suggest, the cultivation of a more positive attitude towards social welfare in general cannot be achieved without respect for diversity. In concrete terms, he draws attention to gender equality problems in the traditional Japanese work-life pattern, which forces men to work long hours and women to stay home. Life is not just about working or only about childrearing, he seems to argue, and he calls for 'diversified values' (p. 146) and a good sense of balance, which make allowances for people's wishes to enjoy their life both at work and outside work, and at home and outside the home, regardless of gender and age.
The epilogues by Wærness and Okazawa interestingly illustrate what they perceive as most wanting in the social welfare system of their respective countries. Even though Norway has relatively well-functioning welfare arrangements in most areas, the care of the elderly is said to be one of the most problematic. Entry into care homes is limited, and there appears to be an unreasonably large amount of pressure placed on the home-help services, a situation that has made the implementation of a *rationality of care* difficult. It should perhaps be pointed out that there is, on the other hand, less need in Norway to emphasize diversity management, as respect for diversity has been one of the most important guiding principles of the Norwegian social welfare state in the past decades.

Reiko Abe Auestad and Yayoi Saito
4th of February, 2010

Acknowledgments

The publication of this book was made possible by a Grant-in-Aid for Publication of Scientific Research Results from the Japan Society for the

Promotion of Science. In addition, the contributors would like to thank all the organizations and people who have supported our research projects over so many years. We would especially like to thank Kyoko Toguchi, adiministrative assistant in the Graduate School of Human Sciences, Osaka University, for her administrative support. Finally We would like to thank Kyoto University Press and their managing director Tetsuya Suzuki, their editor Itaru Saito, Trans Pacific Press and their English-language editor, Cathy Edmonds.

Chapter 1
On the Rationality of Caring

Kari Wærness

Introduction[1]

While rationality has always been a central issue in the social sciences since the time of the founding fathers, caring is a concept that until recent years has scarcely received any attention in sociological literature. What it means to care for others and how care-giving services are to be carried out in the welfare states of the Western world today is now attracting the interest of social scientists; in part, because of the challenges emerging from feminism and the search for a women's perspective in social theory; and, in part, because of the more recent shift in social policy debate dealing with the public services. In Scandinavian countries, for example, public opinion shows a declining confidence in professionalization and socialization, once considered to be the cornerstones in the development of the welfare state. Instead, a belief in so-called *community care* is spreading rapidly because it is supposed to be cheaper and morally preferable to the public care-giving services.

The feminist critique of sociological conceptualizations and theories that do not adequately reflect the position of women in society is highly relevant for understanding this shift or change of direction in social policy thinking. The enthusiasm with which *care by the community* or *informal caring networks* has been discussed in public debate is rarely matched by a clear analysis of either the conditions for, or the consequences of, methods and measures for its implementation. In fact, the knowledge that can be applied to this new policy option is very limited because there are few systematic theories in sociology on the study of reproduction and the social order. There is no conceptual framework that can be applied in analyzing experiences and activities transcending our traditional sociological dichotomies like public/private, home/work, labor/leisure. This makes it difficult to formulate a theory of care-giving work.

Lacking a ready-made conceptual framework, I will use some empirical facts as a starting point to suggest a basis for a more thorough understanding of the factual changes going on in the organization of care-giving work and of the changes in beliefs concerning optimal care giving.

One fundamental fact, of course, is that the responsibility for caring is still ascribed on the basis of gender—as a part of the formation of *femininity*. What this means for women today is that they are faced both with the task of caring for children, the ill, the disabled, and the elderly in the private sphere, while at the same time trying to achieve more command over their own lives and a greater measure of economic independence. The new ideology that informal care is better than public care reinforces these problems (Finch and Groves 1980).

However, the increasing transfer of caring responsibilities from the private sphere has meant that public services have become a very important part of the female labor market. Even if the high-ranking professional and administrative positions in this sector are mostly filled by men, and a great number of the newly created jobs for women are unskilled and low-paid, the importance of the public services for the welfare of working women has to be carefully evaluated.

Such an evaluation seems especially important in a situation where we are confronted with the idea that it would be better to replace these services with different kinds of informal caring. From a woman's perspective, the sociological description of the growth of the public care-giving services as 'an emptying of the functions of the family' or as 'deprivatization of social reproduction' is very inadequate and needs to be re-examined and qualified. In addition to the fact that a lot of research has documented that most of the care-giving work is still performed on a family or private basis (Moroney 1976; Wærness 1978; Sundström 1982), informal resources very often have to be mobilized both to make use of existing social services and to substitute for its shortages. Most often women are the ones who have to cope with the deficiencies of the welfare state services. Besides, many of these services have not first and foremost replaced informal caring, but have instead gradually changed its content, as an increasing number of professional educators, advisors, and consultants have invaded the private sphere (Stacey 1981).

I think the most educated guess that social scientists can offer to the question of community care is the following: any idea of a massive replacement of public services by unpaid and informal caring arrangements is unlikely to be realized in the foreseeable future.[2]

More probably, in societies like ours, the demand for public care will continue to increase as a result of the changes in the age distribution of the population, changes in family behavior, and women's increasing demand for paid employment. Unless more stigma is attached to the use of public services, it also seems reasonable to expect that the number of people who consider public care-giving services to be among the social rights connected with their status as citizens in the welfare state will steadily increase.[3]

As a result of the development of the welfare state, informal care in the private sphere can more adequately be viewed today as a supplement rather than as an alternative to public care. Suggested policy alternatives that aim at transferring more care-giving work from the public to the private sphere already exist and simply need to be activated. This assumption is, however, unrealistic. Social scientists should therefore, first and foremost, concentrate their research and analysis on the possibilities for a more rational use of currently available resources for public care. By *rational* in this context, I mean rational in relation to what most of us in our everyday lives perceive as the essential values in a *caring relationship*.

The recent trend in favor of more community care is, at least in part, a consequence of many people feeling that the public care system lacks the very qualities necessary to transform *services* into *caring*. Both in view of today's economic recession and in view of the challenge posed by those who for reasons other than economic ones question the legitimacy of many welfare state services (Illich 1976), there is a great need to find better models for organizing care-giving work. To develop such models, it seems necessary to study not only the exploitative nature of women's traditional care-giving work, but also the positive qualities inherent in it[4] and why they seem to get lost when it is professionalized and socialized. To be able to carry this analysis further, however, more theoretical attention must first be given to the concept of *caring*.

Caring: labor and feelings

The conceptual and theoretical tools from our sociological tradition are inadequate to analyze a phenomenon like caring. Thus it seems reasonable to use the definition in a well-known dictionary as a starting point. In broad terms, caring is a concept encompassing that range of human experiences that has to do with feeling concern for, and taking charge of, the wellbeing of others. This definition tells us that caring is both about activities and feelings. *Feeling concern* and *taking charge* have both practical and psychological implications. We often choose the words *to care for* to convey a sense of the bonds that tie us to other people in a wide variety of social relationships. We *care for* our friends, our lovers, our children, our parents, our clients, our patients, and sometimes for our neighbors, and even sometimes for people we come into contact with at chance meeting places.

Caring is about relations between (at least two) people.[5] One of them (the carer) shows concern, consideration, affection, devotion, towards the other (the cared for). The one needing care is invaluable to the one providing care, and when the former is suffering pain or discomfort, the latter identifies with her/him and attends to alleviating it. Adult, healthy people feel a need to be cared for by others in many different situations. Worn out, dejected, tired, depressed—there are many adjectives to describe states in which what we need or desire is for others *to care for us*. In such situations we may feel that we have a *right* to our need for care being met. This means there must be others who feel that it is their duty or desire to honor this right. People to whom we are attached through the ties of family, love, or friendship most often are the ones we expect to feel this obligation.

In *principle* caring for healthy adults might be based on equal give-and-take relationships between people who have personal ties to each other. This kind of informal care can be based on *norms of balanced reciprocity* in personal relations; that is, help, support, and favors can be exchanged between people in symmetrical relations. When we say that people *care for each other*, we have this kind of reciprocity in mind. However, as caring first and foremost tends to be associated with women, *much* of the caring that women do for their husbands, older children, and for other adult members of the family does not imply this kind of reciprocity and should therefore, in terms of activities, be defined rather as *personal services*. When women provide these services, it is often something they feel *forced* to do, not out of their concern for the wellbeing of others, but as a result of their subordinate position in the family. When providing help and services to persons who cannot perform these activities themselves—children, the ill, the disabled, the frail elderly—the situation is different. In such relations, the receiver of the care is the subordinate in relation to the caregiver. These groups are dependent on those who feel an obligation or desire to *care for others*.

To provide good care in such relations means that the caregiver at all times performs the activities necessary to satisfy the immediate needs of the cared for. At the same time, most dependents have to meet certain demands and challenges in order to prevent lapses in their development or recovery. Therefore, good caring should be performed in such a way that it, as far as possible, reinforces the self-sufficiency and independence of the receiver. The dependent is to be neither overprotected nor neglected.

Whether we analyze caring as *labor* or as *love*, it seems highly important to make a theoretical distinction between caring for dependents, caring for superiors, and caring in symmetrical relations. Both in emotional and practical terms, it can be assumed that these different categories of caring relations give rise to different problems for women in their struggle for greater independence and autonomy.

These distinctions also make us attentive to problematic situations where women have to choose for whom to care—the weaker or the stronger. Both in women's family roles and in many of the traditional female occupational roles, there is a great risk of confrontations with such dilemmas.[6]

Caring for dependents—that is, those members of society who by normal social standards are unable to take care of themselves—is the field of caring that most clearly is a concern both for social policy and for feminists. In the rest of this chapter I therefore delimit most of the discussion to problems connected with caring for dependents, involving people who take on active caring on a consistent and reliable basis. This kind of caring I define as care-giving work, whether it is paid or unpaid, no matter whether it takes place in the public or in the private sphere.

Reproduction becomes a science

The traditional arguments for ascribing caring functions to women, in addition to the unquestionable fact that only women give birth to children, are founded on a perception of women as more intuitive and emotional than men. With the modernization of society, however, this ascribed *natural inclination* was no longer assumed to be sufficient for women to become *good* carers, either in the private or in the public sphere. In addition, they needed to acquire *some* formal knowledge based on science. Scientific work, however, was not for women. Either they were considered to be intellectually incapable of doing research, or scientific work was assumed to be detrimental to their biological function. (It is interesting to note that no one seems to have argued that it is *illogical* that only members of the gender not qualified for practicing care should be capable of giving expert advice on how it should be carried out.) We also find explicitly stated, if not so often, that the defining criterion of scientific knowledge—objectivity—is essentially masculine. For example, George Simmel (cited in List 1983: 6) writes:

> The requirement—of correctness in practical judgment and objectivity in theoretical knowledge—belong as it were in their form and their claims to humanity in general, but in their actual historical configuration they are masculine throughout. Supposing that we describe these things, viewed as absolute ideas, by the single word 'objective', we then find that in the history of our race the equation objective = masculine is a valid one.

The scientification of reproductive work, which in the Scandinavian countries started in the second part of the nineteenth century, meant that women became subordinated to a new kind of male authority—the authority of scientific knowledge. On the one hand the emergence of this new kind of authority meant a substitution or a decline of other kinds of authority—the authority of the husband/father and of the clerical profession. On the other hand, this scientification also implied that women lost positions of authority and control. The increasing power of the medical profession, still the most authoritative in the field of reproduction, is the most important case in this respect. The traditional lay healthcare system consisted of autonomous healers of both sexes, and the whole field of pregnancy and childbirth belonged to the female sphere. The history of midwifery, which is somewhat different in various Western countries, tells us that the increasing influence of doctors everywhere led to midwives losing status and autonomy (Ehrenreich and English 1973; Oakley 1976). At the same time, the medical profession's control over healthcare created new subordinate roles for women. Both mothers and nurses became medical auxiliaries, executing what the doctors prescribed (Donzelot 1979: 7–49).

Much research has documented how this increasing scientific control over reproduction should not be described as an unambiguous development of progress and humanization. In the fields of obstetrics, childcare, health, psychiatry, and care for the mentally retarded and so on—everywhere—we find examples of professionals at times confounding traditional practices (which the experts of later times evaluate as better than the ones their predecessors prescribed) on the basis of 'what we know from science.'[7] The same has been true for domestic activities such as keeping house, cooking, and cleaning. Textbooks on domestic science and infant care written by male doctors and published in Norway during the past hundred years clearly give the impression of a belief in the omnipotence of science and the impotence of women, even if the latter belief is not explicitly stated in the more recent books. An illustrative example of this can be found in Norwegian history at the time when the first attempt to make housewifery into a domestic science was made.

The first two textbooks on housewifery based on scientific knowledge, published in Norway about 1860, were followed by a great public debate among members of the male elite about the quality of women's work in the household. Some years earlier a woman, Hanna Winsnes, had started to write such textbooks, based not on scientific knowledge but on her practical experiences as a housewife in a large bourgeois family household for more than forty years. Comparing her books with the *scientific* ones, the modesty of Hanna Winsnes sharply contrasts with the arrogance of the male authors. Only in the textbook intended to be of special help to the poorest housewives does she moralize in an authoritarian manner. On the basis of today's accepted standards for good practices, however, Hanna Winsnes's books still excel over those written by male scientists. Many of her recipes, for instance, even if too bothersome for modern housewives, *could* still be used with relatively good results for a healthy and palatable diet.

The same does not hold for the scientific books. Their recipes are mostly too inaccurate to be of much help to the inexperienced cook, and many of their general recommendations are the reverse of what is considered to be correct according to current standards. The male authors use much space to argue, in a very arrogant style, why women's traditional practices (including those of Hanna Winsnes) are basically wrong, suggesting that women therefore need some formal knowledge in order to be better housewives. Notwithstanding the praise they received from their contemporary critics, these scientific textbooks were soon forgotten. Hanna Winsnes's books, on the other hand, in spite of much criticism from the male elite, sold thousands of copies over a period of more than fifty years.

The recommendations of experts in the field of childcare, on subjects ranging from breast- and bottle-feeding, toilet-training, weaning, eating, and sleeping, to more general problems of discipline and punishment, have also changed very much over time. To a certain extent it has also been found that what experts considered the only right thing to do at one time, they later consider totally wrong. Whatever the content of the advice, however, it has often been expressed in such an authoritative manner that a mother who does not manage to follow it may get the impression that she will permanently harm her children.

Evaluating the present state of knowledge on this subject, John and Elizabeth Newson (1976: 14) admit that:

> there is not a sufficient body of well-substantiated evidence about the facts and consequences of child rearing on which to base sound practical advice to parents. There is no lack of theoretical speculation, but so far very few theories of child rearing have been subjected to the inconvenience of being reconciled with the empirical evidence. Whatever the reason may be for this unfortunate state of affairs, the situation can hardly have arisen simply because the subject has no importance: indeed, it is probably because it has such immense importance that the professional advisers and pseudo-experts have flourished in such profusion.

As some professionals in recent years have become more modest in their roles as advisers, the arguments for the necessity of *parents' education* have shifted. As science has documented the importance and value of some of the traditional practices that earlier were denounced, parents' education is now seen as necessary because of the assumed decline of the extended family and increasing lack of informal caring networks.[8] In addition to the more modest experts, we still have professionals believing in the omnipotence of science. Schaffer (1977: 11) seems to be one of them:

> There is, in fact, no reason why bringing up the under-fives should not also be guided by firm knowledge scientifically established rather than depend, as happens at present, on fashion, prejudice and what grandmother says. The parent-child relationship need be no more immune from properly conducted objective inquiry than the movements of the planets or the structure of DNA—even if its analysis presents problems of far greater complexity.

We have very little factual information on how mothers react to the experts' different and often contradictory recommendations. However, the number of experts invading the private sphere has steadily increased, and women's formal training in school and employment teaches them to act according to the dominant kinds of rationality in the public sphere. The question of whether this is counterproductive to their developing the skills and attitudes necessary for *rational care giving* therefore becomes important. Most mothers today probably agree with the scientific experts that natural inclination is not sufficient to handle the problems they face in caring for their children. How much help they receive from formal knowledge and professional advice, however, is an unanswered question. The studies of Oakley (1974) and Holter et al. (1967)[9] support the assumption that the conclusions of Lopata (1971), based on a study of American metropolitan housewives, holds for Western women in general.

> The social role of mother does not produce many women who express full confidence in their ability to perform it at desired levels. In fact, the more educated the American metropolitan woman, the more conscious she is of the complexity of this role and of the difficulties involved in competent child-rearing. The relational emphasis of this type of mother, combined with a societal focusing of responsibility on her and awareness of the importance of the home for child development, make for worry over actions designed to best meet the goals of the relation. The physical care of an offspring is no longer a major source of concern, as it was for the lower-class antecedents of the modern woman; she

> quite competently handles preventative and curative situations of child health. It is her desire to provide the offspring with the best available resources for the development of their personality and potentials, coupled with the inadequacy of the sources of knowledge which she can utilize, which creates the greatest degree of concern for the new American woman (Lopata 1971: 375–6).

That more theoretical knowledge does not always improve the quality of care-giving work should not lead us to the conclusion that less knowledge would be better. Instead, we have to ask *what kind* of knowledge is relevant in order to deal with problems that cannot be mastered by finding the perfect techniques or by acting according to bureaucratic rules, but where the quality of the work still depends on the actors' training and skills.

Wittgenstein (cited in McMillan 1982: 41–2), when discussing a somewhat different problem in *Philosophical Investigations,* illuminates what also seems to be a crucial problem when discussing notions of learning and teaching in the context of care giving.

> Is there such a thing as "expert judgement" about the genuineness of expressions of feeling?...Even here, there are those whose judgement is "better" and those whose judgement is "worse".
>
> Correcter prognoses will generally issue from the judgements of those with better knowledge of mankind.
>
> Can one learn this knowledge? Yes: some can. *Not, however, by taking a course in it, but through "experience"*...Can someone else be a man's teacher in this? Certainly. From time to time he gives him the right tip. This is what "learning" and "teaching" are like here...*What one acquires is not a technique; one learns correct judgements.* There are also rules, but they do not form a system, and *only experienced people can apply* them right. Unlike calculating rules.
>
> What is most difficult here is to put this indefiniteness, correctly and unfalsified, into words (emphases added).

To the extent that scientific knowledge becomes an absolute gauge of what counts as knowledge, Wittgenstein reminds us that this can be detrimental to practices that earlier belonged to the non-scientific sphere. In the realm of care giving, where we have a long tradition of male scientific arrogance in evaluating women's practices, this problem today seems to be highly relevant.

The ambivalence with which women writers confront the phenomenon *science* is probably not only a result of the continuing exclusion of women from the business of science. I agree with List (1983) that the roots of this ambivalence go deeper. It is also because of personal experience that, until recently, a feminist critique of the social sciences was seldom clearly articulated. Science's rationalist culture, and the models of behavior that it propagates, are contradictory, if not hostile, to the feelings that women see as their own. A central task of feminist research, in my opinion, then, is to look at the context of care-giving work and evaluate the use of conventional scientific concepts and models, which may well account for the fact that important problems remain overlooked. Furthermore, in this field, female social scientists can use their personal experiences from everyday life to suggest alternative models. These alternatives can contribute to change in social theory and research, which will better reflect the realities and interests of both women and the weakest members of society. A new image of the social actor and a reconceptualization of *rationality* emerging from women's studies seem to be a promising starting point.

The sentient actor and the rationality of caring

Both on the basis of my personal experiences of care giving in the private sphere and from my empirical research on care-giving work, I find it reasonable to argue the following: there exists something that should be called *the rationality of caring*, which is of fundamental importance for the welfare of dependents, and at the same time different from and to some degree contradictory to the scientific rationality on which professional authority and control in the field of reproduction is legitimated. Titmuss (1963: 126) verges on this problem when he writes about the patients' situation in the modern hospital:

> Why is it not understood that courtesy and sociability have a therapeutic value? *Most of us in our home know this instinctively, but somehow or other it gets lost in the hospital* (emphasis added).

Apart from the fact that courtesy and sociability are probably of greater importance in situations where therapy no longer has any effect, one important reason that this knowledge is forgotten could be that the value of kindness and politeness cannot be calculated. I further disagree with Titmuss that we know anything about caring *by instinct*. In some way or another it has to be learned. Even if emotions are important for our caring for others in the private sphere, it seems evident that the ability to care in a *proper* way depends on something that can be learned and for which there are rules for proceeding, and that therefore some kind of rationality is involved.

To accept a conceptualization like *the rationality of caring* is to go against the mainstream of Western philosophy and sociology, which deals with rationality and emotionality (or instrumentality and expressiveness) as two mutually exclusive qualities of human action—a mainstream that traditionally has defined women as less rational human beings than men. Weber (1966), for instance, even if arguing that emotions are important, still posits a model of social action that defines action based on emotion, like action based on ignorance and tradition, as nonrational.[10] This raises two problems: a confusion between rationality and lack of emotion, and the implication that emotions and feelings are not positively required by the rational action of individuals or by the smooth functioning of institutions (Hochschild 1975: 284).

In the normal discourse of everyday reasoning, however, this dualistic image of rationality and emotionality is not always self-evident. Most people probably experience emotions and feelings as active and legitimate ingredients in behavior, which they, at the same time, define as rational.

A renowned dictionary does not support the assumption of the mutual exclusiveness of emotionality and rationality, showing that it has not been totally accepted in our everyday language. According to *Webster's New World Dictionary* (1976), one definition of *rational* is the following: 'The ability to reason logically as by drawing conclusions from inferences and *often* connotes the absence of emotionalism.' To assume that some kind of rationality is also operating in activities and relations where emotions are of crucial importance, therefore, does not seem idiosyncratic according to how rationality *can* be interpreted in everyday life, even in a rationalized culture like ours.

Russell Hochschild (1975) argues that we need a new image of the social actor in addition to the two images that hitherto have dominated much of the social sciences. The first image is that of the *conscious, cognitive actor*. This image portrays people as consciously wanting something (e.g. money and status) and consciously calculating the merit of various means to reach this end. The second image, indebted to Freud, is that of the *unconscious, emotional actor*. Here the actor is guided by unconscious motivations and does and thinks things whose meanings are better understood by the social scientist than by the actor. As Hochschild points out, these two images do not *deny* affective consciousness; images deny nothing.

However, it is a commonplace insight of the sociology of knowledge that we collectively construct social reality, that what we define as real is real. Because of the authority, prestige, and influence of scientific institutions in modern society, science not only describes but also prescribes social situations and forms of social actions. So, if we believe that, for instance, the scientific understanding that head and heart, or emotions and rationality, are antithetical, we act on the basis of this definition and organize our lives so as to confirm this belief. Our experience then provides evidence that our definition is correct and the duality goes on and on. It therefore seems important to include in the social sciences an image of a social actor who is *both* conscious and feeling. Russell Hochschild suggests *the sentient actor* as a third image necessary to remind social scientists that human actors must be seen as more than bloodless calculators or blind expressers of uncontrolled emotions. In order to analyze phenomena like caring and care giving, which seem to fall in a no-man's land when we focus either on the conscious cognitive actor or the unconscious emotional actor, this image of the sentient actor seems adequate.[11] Further, this image gives meaning to a conceptualization like *the rationality of caring.*

To arrive at a better understanding of how the rationality of caring differs from scientific rationality, we can analyze how *learning* in the context of motherly care, as an ideal type in the Weberian sense, differs from *learning* in the context of science. In the context of science, one understands from the position of an outsider, and learning means to develop the ability to formulate a body of principles based on what is common to many phenomena and therefore independent of the peculiar and individual. One learns from books and theories and shows that one knows something by being able to subsume the important points in a neat system of laws. In science, one searches for predictability and control, the dominant criteria according to which scientific success is measured.

In the context of motherly care one has to think and act on the level of the particular and individual. This means one has to understand from the position of an insider, and the kind of generalized scientific knowledge one may have, at best, seems very insufficient in guiding one's practices. Moreover, 'as the child grows it requires different things from its mother and this means that she can never perfect her techniques, but must remain flexible and capable of adapting to a changed situation' (Kitzinger 1978: 34). Or, in the words of McMillan (1982: 54):

> It is vital for mothers to be aware that there are many things in life which can neither be learned from books nor understood from the position of an outsider. It is only because we realize that acting with rigid consistency is not always a sign of reasonable and appropriate behaviour that we do not think a mother is stupid when for example, we see her from one day to the next, making delicate adjustments in the care of her infant which other people would not think worthwhile.

The point, which all of those who advocate standardizing and making scientific our methods of childrearing seem to miss, is the following: in the context of everyday life, it is foolish to seek *certainty* in one's personal relations. The aim to provide women with scientific certainty that their method of childrearing will be successful is pseudo-science, because the relation between individuals is, by definition, something that cannot be subsumed under any kind of statistical generalization. Once that is done, the aspect of individuality vanishes.

It is therefore not surprising that mothers seem to be extremely hesitant about concocting theories about how other people should bring up their children, and that many of them are still skeptical about the advice thrust upon them by *experts*.

Expertise in childrearing, according to the rationality of caring, is dependent both on practical experience in care-giving work and on personal knowledge of the individual child in question. When mothers exchange advice and support concerning problems of childcare, they can therefore at the same time insist that it is easier to bring up the second child than the first, and still say that each child has to be treated quite differently. To search for the kind of precision inherent in scientific rationality therefore seems foolish or wrong in the context of care giving.

To illustrate the point of how working according to the rules of scientific rationality in some contexts can be counterproductive to what could be defined as rational behavior, the work of a cook can be compared with the work of a chemist:

> The use of a chemical balance in her kitchen would not make an inferior cook a better one because in the kitchen the role that the accuracy of measurements plays is not comparable with its importance in a chemistry experiment. For example, while it is obviously important to mix the ingredients in the right proportion if a good cake is to be made, it is possible to juggle with them in order to obtain a certain effect in a way that would be quite unacceptable in an experiment. Moreover the reasons why someone may be a bad cook, in contradistinction to being a bad chemist, may have nothing to do with inaccurate measurements.
>
> *In some cases it may actually result from following a recipe rigidly and not knowing how to adapt it to suit one's own particular tastes and circumstances. Such knowledge, however, depends on practice and on the help* of those *who are experienced cooks* (McMillan 1982: 49; emphasis added).

These arguments about concrete activities like cooking may seem trivial or obvious, at least on the level of everyday reasoning.[12] In planning public care-giving services, a similar attitude to the importance of personal knowledge and a lack of rigidity should be considered reasonable, or rational. To the extent that such evaluations should be taken into account, it follows that professional and bureaucratic control has to be diminished. As the professionalization and bureaucratization of the public care system still seem to be increasing, this tells us that such evaluations may be contradictory to the principles upon which the whole ideology of public planning is based, and therefore not so easy to implement.

From various empirical studies of different public care-giving services, however, it seems that the image of the sentient actor is a perfectly adequate one in order to understand the behavior and attitudes of the caregivers in the lower positions in organizational hierarchies (Abrahamsson and Söder 1977; Liljeström and Özgalda 1980; Ressner 1981; Viklund 1981). The same image emerges from my own study of home helps (Wærness 1982: 136–80). The work of these home helps was organized in such a way that the individual employee provided flexible and versatile services and help to a few clients over longer periods of time. The most satisfying feature of these home help jobs was said to be their personal attachment to the clients. In fact, this aspect seemed to be the main reason why they felt happy about their jobs and wanted to stick to them. These middle-aged and elderly women argued that their experiences as housewives in their own families for many years was the most important training for being able to do a good job as a home help. Even those who had special formal training for this occupation doubted it had any value, apart from heightening the status of their job.[13] Working on the basis of their competence as housewives, however, often meant they had to break the official job instructions. Often they had to work for more hours than they were paid, and sometimes they even had to do things that were directly forbidden according to the rules. They also expressed a very clear opinion about the negative aspects of their work. The isolated working situation, which meant they had no colleagues to share problems and experiences with, and the lack of influence compared to the more professionalized working groups in the social services, were regarded as very negative features of their work role. They also had a very clear understanding that their conduct as employees in many ways could be evaluated as foolish according to the general norms for rational behavior in the labor market. Still, they gave priority to doing what seemed right according to the rationality of caring.

Public authorities feel compelled today to change the current organization of the home help service; in part, to secure the individual home help the same rights as other employees in the labor market and, in part, because of the diminishing supply of middle-aged housewives who are both willing and feel competent to work under the same conditions as in the past. The authorities admit that it may be difficult to find measures to change the organization without changing the service in such a way that it becomes less personal and comprehensive.

In their study about wards in institutions for the mentally retarded, Abrahamsson and Söder (1977) used flexibility in work as an indicator of 'good caring'. The work was said to be flexible to the extent that the behavior of the staff varied over time and in relation to the individualized needs of the mentally retarded person involved (Söder 1981: 48). To be capable of working in this way, I assume the individual caregiver had to be both conscious and feeling (i.e. *a sentient actor*). In investigating the relationships between flexibility in work and different organizational characteristics of the institutions, this study shows that decentralization of power was the factor most strongly correlated with flexibility in work. Wards where the staff had influence over decisions relevant to their work functioned with greater flexibility than wards where decision-making powers were centralized. The way work was coordinated was also found to be of importance. Wards where work was coordinated by formal planning and detailed instructions were often working in a routinized, non-flexible way. More access to experts of any kind, a remedy that planning authorities generally believe is for the better, showed no direct correlation with the degree of flexibility in work. Still more importantly, it could be shown that a more professionally trained staff did not result in more flexibility. On the contrary, formal training seemed to promote a tendency to more routinization, a finding so surprising in relation to accepted truths that it needed further comment:

> It must be reasonable to assume that increased knowledge on the part of the staff should lead to more flexibility at the workplace. When we still do not find more flexibility on wards with a high proportion of educated personnel, we have to question the content of the education. Only to insist that education is for the good, seems meaningless as long as one does not specify what kind of knowledge the caregivers need (Abrahamsson and Söder 1977: 80).

One explanation for the fact that professional training did not further flexibility could be that this kind of learning socializes individuals to think and act according to the values inherent in scientific rationality and in such a way that the values inherent in the rationality of caring become degraded or suppressed. In other words, the conscious cognitive actor becomes more of an ideal than the sentient actor. Because the head–heart duality is accepted in all sciences, it seems probable that any kind of formal education based on scientific knowledge will to some degree promote a more instrumental attitude towards work, at the expense of the expressive.

What studies of medical education say about this problem probably has some relevance for most formal education in the field of care giving. Merton and Barber (1967) describe the doctor's role as one of 'detached concern.' They refer to the combination of detachment (an instrumental trait) and concern (an expressive trait) as a perfect example of sociological ambivalence in that it involves an oscillation between conflicting norms:

> the therapist role of the physician...calls for *both* a degree of affective detachment for the patient and a degree of compassionate concern for him... Since these norms cannot be *simultaneously* expressed in behaviour, they come to be expressed in an *oscillation* of behaviours: of detachment and compassion, of discipline and permissiveness, of personal and impersonal treatment (Merton and Barber 1967: 96; emphases added).

To the degree that formal education for caregivers in subordinate positions also leads to a strengthening of the belief in the duality of rationality and emotion, this can explain why the educated caregivers become less able or willing to give individualized care than the ones with no formal training at all.[14] Changes in the work roles of nurses support this view. In trying to achieve professional and academic status, leading nurses everywhere tend to favor the development of formally acquired knowledge. This one-sidedness has led to a devaluation of the informally acquired and intuitive kind of knowledge and skills that are learned through practicing bedside care (Alvsvag 1981; Martinsen and Wærness 1979). More *nursing science* is therefore not a solution to the problem of strengthening the values inherent in the rationality of caring, at least as long as this science is based on the generally accepted notions of scientific knowledge and learning.

Schumacher argues that there are many problems in human life that cannot be solved through scientific reasoning, but where such reasoning instead leads to different answers that appear to be the exact opposites (Schumacher 1978). These types of problems he proposes to call *divergent* problems in contrast to *convergent* problems to which the scientific methodology of problem solving is adequate. Most of the examples of divergent problems he mentions belong to the realm of care giving. What he argues about divergent problems in general therefore seems to have great relevance for the problems emerging from the increasing professionalization of care-giving work.

> Divergent problems offend the logical mind which wishes to remove tension by coming down on one side or the other; but they provoke, stimulate and sharpen the higher human faculties without which man is nothing but a clever animal. A refusal to accept the divergency of divergent problems causes these higher faculties to remain dormant and to wither away, and when this happens the "clever animal" is more likely than not to destroy itself.
>
> Man's life can thus be seen and understood as a succession of divergent problems which are inevitably encountered and have to be coped with in some way. They are refractory to mere logic and discursive reason, and constitute, as it were, a strain-and-stretch apparatus to develop the Whole Man, and that means to develop man's supra-logical faculties. All traditional cultures have seen life as a school and have recognized, in one way or another, the essentiality of this teaching force (Schumacher 1978: 147–8).

Better care giving: a question of finding new principles for organisation

Scientific rationality is related to people's fundamental need for autonomy and control and has constantly celebrated new victories as more and more spheres of life in modern society have become rationalized. At the same time, this rationalization has meant that other fundamental human needs, above all the need for care and closeness—needs we have learned to label *feminine*—have become devalued. In order to be real persons, with self-respect and worthy of the esteem of others, modern men have to define themselves as *independent.* That 'there is an element of dependence in every relationship, even with a dog,' as Freud expressed it, and the fact that helplessness and dependency are part of life itself for all of us—in childhood, illness, and old age—may in part be hidden and repressed as long as the caring function is left to an invisible, oppressed women's culture. Still, women provide most of the care-giving work as unpaid family work and the bulk of the helping that in Western societies is reported as community care turns out, on closer scrutiny, to be care by close female relatives, a point that is seldom clearly stated (Abrams 1977).

As women to an increasing degree have become socialized to the dominant values in a rationalized society, their 'dual-life' in the 'welfare-service society' not only implies a heavy daily workload; it also means that they have to cope with the antithetical expectations of instrumentalism and expressiveness (Glennon 1979: 160–4). This coping is the more difficult as these dual expectations are present *both* in women's family roles and most of their paid work roles.

It seems reasonable to assume that the scientification of reproduction has had an independent effect on most women's feelings of insecurity and lack of competence in all kinds of care giving in the private sphere, whether they are well integrated in an informal female network or not. This is a point that many advocates for more community care as a solution to the crisis in the public care system seem to miss. As Stacey and Price (1981: 100–32) have pointed out, the autonomy of women in the domestic sphere has gradually been so reduced that younger women today scarcely have a private domain in which they feel able and competent. Today's emphasis on more community care as a basis for a hierarchical and professionalized public care system, to the extent that it could at all be realized, would therefore most probably lead to professional caregivers working as advisers and consultants being strengthened, and still more of the practical tasks being left to subordinate and unpaid female members of the family. Furthermore, the development of non-stigmatizing public services in the welfare state has been shown to be important for dependent people in order for them to maintain a kind of balanced reciprocity in their family relations. When they have access to such services, the chances are greater that they can be on good, affectionate terms with their family members and receive help and support from them, which they value very positively, because they are not totally dependent on them (Nordhus 1981).

Research from different countries shows that the wish to maintain what Rosenmayr and Köckeis (1965) call 'intimacy—but at a distance' describes the kind of relation a growing number of aged people prefer to have with their children (Shanas 1979). A wish to maintain 'intimacy—but at a distance' seems to be a typical attitude among the aged and disabled, not only in the area of family relations, but in relation to the public care system as well. The popularity of the home help system (i.e. a care-giving service that moves on the borderline between the domestic and the public sphere and is very little professionalized) may be an indication of this development.

Studies of women's self-organized care-giving work on *the hidden market* also show that care-giving work can be paid. At the same time much importance can be attached to ensuring that the relation between provider and receiver is to be comprehensive, personal, and characterized by equality (Gullestad 1984). We also know that clients can prefer to have their daughters or daughters-in-law as home helps, paid by the social services. On the other hand, nonrelated home helps can be regarded as 'daughters' or 'friends' (Schorr 1962: 419; Teeland 1978: 170–1). Such attitudes towards combining personal attachment and payment in a relation are mainly found among working-class women.[15] Middle-class women are more likely to regard the paid care-giving relations also on the hidden market more in terms of a contractual employer–employee relation.[16]

When people therefore deplore payment of informal care giving on the grounds that the introduction of market values damages the quality of care, this is a typical middle-class evaluation. Both in the private and the public sphere, much of the paid care giving of working-class women, both today and in earlier times, contradicts this evaluation. On the other hand, not all kinds of private and unpaid care are of *good quality*. When focusing on the problems of today's public services as being too impersonal, rigid, and intensive, it is easy to forget the problems of oppression, injustice, violence, abuse, and moralizing, which can arise in more private and personalized caring relations. When public authorities today appear to accept the idea that the care for those who mainly need human consideration, warmth, and a bit more time[17] is better left to voluntary organizations than to the public care system, they seem to have forgotten the working-class historical experiences with voluntary work in the form of charity.

However, the greatest problem within the public care system today is that there is too much detachment, not that there is too much concern. From the little evidence that exists, *more concern*, in fact, is not primarily a question of whether care giving is being paid or not.

Strengthening the values inherent in the rationality of caring is, therefore, in today's welfare state, not a question of replacing public *paid* care with informal *unpaid* family care or voluntary work. Rather, it seems to be a question of what possibilities there are to recognize the public care system in such a way that practical experience in care-giving work and personal knowledge of the individual client can be an independent basis for greater influence, at the expense of professional and bureaucratic control and authority.

As virtually all prophets—or as they are now called, futurologists—seem to agree that the future will see an ever increasing reliance on specialized knowledge and skill and on applying that knowledge to the solution of practical problems by specially trained men (Bell 1968), such a change may seem rather utopian. Freidson (1973) argues that the tendency towards the work of many other occupations in the different organizations to be coordinated around a professionalized service would increase in the future. Post-industrial society, in his opinion, will be the professional society.

However, the growing skepticism in recent years about further professionalization as a means of solving the ills of the capitalistic welfare state may imply that there is a chance that this trend could be counteracted.

Some representatives of the prestigious medical profession also admit that 'the time has come for a major conceptual shift in the health care policy debate, from viewing lay people as consumers of health care to seeing them as they really are: its primary providers' (Levin and Idler 1981: 1), so there may be reason to be optimistic. Further, in the face of the substantial shift in the pattern of diseases in the Western world over the past forty years, from approximately 30% of all diseases being chronic to the present 80%[18] (a shift that the medical delivery system has been unable to adjust to adequately), the need for change seems urgent.

For a greater limitation or diminution of professional and bureaucratic control in the public services to be possible, there is a need for a fundamental change in the values of the interpretational frameworks of the public administration and the political bodies; an acknowledgment that many of the problems in the public care system today are *divergent* problems that cannot be *solved* with any kind of scientific methodology, but that still must be *coped with* on the basis of human actors' knowledge and skills.

More decision-making power to women on the basis of their personal experiences from practical care-giving work in the private sphere and from working-class jobs in the public care-giving services seems at least to be a necessary condition for this to be realized.

Using Dawe's metaphor of sociology as a conversation in which the prime imperative is that 'we ceaselessly listen to and converse with the voices from everyday life...including our own' (Dawe 1988: 414), a feminist sociology could be a tool to visualize how concrete reforms in the public care system could further such changes, and thereby strengthen the values inherent in the rationality of caring.

From what we already know, the organizational principle on which we should insist, in order to improve the situation both for dependents and caregivers today, could be worded like this: 'Small, but not too small, is beautiful.' This means that neither the small, private, and intimate family nor the highly professionalized and specialized public care system provide the kind of flexible and comprehensive care that seems optimal in relation to both dependents' and caregivers' contradictory needs for both autonomy and closeness.

Chapter 2
Between Late Modern and Later Modern Elderly Care in Norway and Japan

Karen Christensen

Introduction

From a Japanese perspective the Scandinavian countries are often seen as generous welfare states with well-developed services for their citizens. This is due to the fact that the public within these countries, generally seen, takes a considerable part of the responsibility for the citizen's welfare. If we place Japan and Norway into a spectrum of different welfare states across the world (Esping-Andersen 1990, 1999), this picture seems to be confirmed. In this spectrum Norway belongs to the cluster of social democratic welfare states, represented first and foremost by the Scandinavian countries. This model implies extended social rights, little private provision, and universalism, which means that the services cover the working class as well as the middle class. On the contrary, today's Japan most likely would be placed in the cluster of conservative welfare states because the state takes only limited responsibility for a citizen's welfare and maintains the role of the family as a central contributor to the care of elderly people.

Here, I want to refine and concretize this general picture of Norway as a very generous welfare state, in contrast with a limited welfare state like Japan, using elderly care as a case. On one hand, I want to do this by giving an overview of the development of elderly care in Norway and, by that, showing that even Norway has some dark sides within its welfare state. On the other hand I want to discuss some of the current Japanese solutions to elderly care in relation to the Norwegian ones and, through this, indicate fundamental differences, as well as some similarities, between these two welfare systems. In general, I aim to present elderly care as resulting from social political intentions, dominating cultural ideologies, and specific country characteristics.

Modernization

The concept of *modernization* is my central tool for analyzing elderly care in this chapter. It means that I will look at the development undergone by the welfare state as a process of modernization, including different stages. In everyday speech, modernization is often coded as a positive word. It is supposed to be something that is improving things and making them more effective. However, in this chapter I want to use a sociological version of this concept. Theories about modernity have been major and ongoing inspirations in sociological thinking since the first general sociological ideas came into being. And many sociologists point to modernity as one of the main subjects of sociology. The difference between *modernity* and *modernization* is reflected in the difference between a status or position and a process. Thus, modernity is the final stage of a certain kind of modernization.

When it comes to the social historical roots of pointing at modernity as a main sociological subject, there are different views of why this is so. First, the view I prefer is the one pointing at the 'two great revolutions' of eighteenth- and nineteenth-century Europe (Giddens 1982). While the first one is the French Revolution of 1789, the second one is the industrial revolution, usually traced back to Britain in the late-eighteenth century. The general inspirations coming from these great revolutions are, on the one hand, the ideas of liberty and democracy, and, on the other hand, the social revolutions, which in this case concern the enormous social and economic changes following the transition from agrarian production to city-based industrial production. However, while these roots are general historical roots to the analysis of modernity throughout times, different areas of society will develop different kinds of modernization. Thus, the modernization of elderly care has to be analyzed on the basis of conditions relevant to this specific area of society. But the tools with which to do it can fruitfully be inspired by general sociological ideas. Thus, in my view, the sociological version of modernization supplies the everyday concept of this phenomenon with a critical view, with a perspective from which to look at it, and with an effort to base the statements on analytical investigations. The critical view implies that the development has to be confronted with questions about, for example, the development's impact on equality and democracy. In other words, a sociological perspective on modernization requires critical and challenging questions. Second, the perspective I want to use is a historical perspective (Abrams 1982) in order to understand elderly care as a continuously developing phenomenon. And, third, the statements in this chapter are based on my own empirical-based care research, as well as on contributions from other care researchers.

In the following section I introduce an overview of the modernization of Norwegian home-based elderly care and relate this overview to the Japanese case.

A short—and even shorter—history of public elderly care

Public home care services in Norway have their earliest roots in the 1960s. However, a public service did not really develop until the 1970s. And since then there have been large changes in the services. On the basis of research into Norwegian home care services, I will investigate this process as a development that can be broken down into three phases of modernization called *traditional care*, *modern services*, and *late modern outputs* (Christensen 2005).[1]

Roughly speaking, the three phases of modernization correspond to the three decades of the 1970s, 1980s, and 1990s, although certain characteristics of one phase may well originate in the foregoing phase and the last phase continues into the 2000s. In general, Norway founded its welfare state following the Second World War, and it has since been progressively developed. And this development has led to important basic changes in the relationships between four different providers in the field of elderly care: the state, the market, the family, and the voluntary sector. Home care has its roots in voluntary (unpaid) work organized by women's organizations in Oslo in the 1950s, but it took seventeen years before the state began to subsidize it, which it did in 1969 (Wærness 1982). Subsequently, home help became increasingly successful, and its activities were expanded. By the 1970s Norway had become a typical Scandinavian welfare state. As such, it embodied a high degree of universalism and assumed considerable responsibility for the social welfare of its citizens, which means that it provided services not just to the working class but also to the middle classes. In the 1980s this picture began to change. Certain kinds of services were cut back, and ideologies were developed to legitimate the reductions. By the 1990s it had become clear that the welfare state no longer assumed all the responsibilities it had taken on in the 1970s and 1980s. Many of these responsibilities were transferred back to the individual, which in practice often meant the individual's female relatives. The changes also entailed greater involvement of the private sector, which in this context encompasses everything from informal family networks and voluntary organizations to commercially provided services.

Although the history of public elderly care in Norway is relatively short, starting in the 1960s, the Japanese history is much shorter. If we take the Long-Term Care Insurance System as the starting point for public elderly care services in Japan, we are talking about a corresponding period beginning in the year 2000. A forerunner of this insurance system was, however, the Gold Plan from 1989. This plan was a ten-year strategy to promote health care and social services for elderly people until the year 2000 by increasing the numbers of home helpers and day service centers. But this was not a comprehensive plan like the new long-term system (see Chapter 3). The Long-Term Care Insurance System has made people sixty-five years and older eligible to receive care services by paying 10% of the actual cost. People are assessed for their eligibility for different levels of help. The system includes eight levels, starting with a level of not needing help (being 'independent'); the next level is 'requiring support 1–2'; and the highest level of help is care level 5 (in the group 'care level 1–5'). People on level 5 are usually bedridden or have dementia and require long-term care. The system offers home-based care, care in institutions (except for those on the lowest level), day services, and assistive technology; some of these services depend on the local municipality conditions. Priority is particularly given in this new system to improving home care services.

The state finances 25% of this system; another 25% is financed by the municipalities, 40% by citizens aged forty and over, and the last 10% is financed by the users of the services. The explanation for including younger citizens, although they are not expected to be dependent on public care, is financial. Presumably, the expenses of the system make this necessary. Compared to the tax-based welfare system in Norway, the Japanese system is different from this as it only covers half of its system through public funding, while covering the other half by insurance directly paid by the users and potential users. However, in Norway people who have been allocated home care services pay an income-based user payment, while nursing services are provided free of charge. Although Norway includes a user payment, it does not run an insurance-based system like the Japanese one. However, while it could be questioned whether there really are fundamental differences concerning this financial aspect—and more of such aspects will be mentioned below—there is a fundamental cultural difference in the basis for the welfare when it comes to family relations.

The fundamental difference can be reflected in the following ideas about the family. While in Norway family relations are maintained by reducing the duties of support given by children to their parents, the Japanese idea, on the contrary, seems to be that good family relations are maintained by the duty of support given to the family's elderly members. Thus, this Japanese family ideology also includes the idea of preferring family members to strangers as care providers. Historical roots for this Japanese ideology can be found in the Meiji Civil Law (1887–1947) and the Imperial Educational Edict (see Saito 2002 and Edvardsen 2005). The Meiji Civil Law gave the oldest son of the family the duty to take care of the family's elderly members, although the care was often provided by the daughter-in-law. Compliance with this law and the Imperial Educational Edict demands support of parents by their children until the parents die. Following this law and imperial edict, a strong moral and ethical duty to take care of the family was established throughout time in Japan. Thus, in 1996 more than 30% of Japanese people still thought that the support of elderly people is a natural duty for children (Saito 2002: 199). It is likely that the number would be even higher if it was not for the Public Assistance Law, implemented in 1956, which announced the right to a healthy and culturally rich life for everybody. At the same time, a new housing system changed the tradition of several generations living together and encouraged nuclear family life. Furthermore, there are several demographic and social explanations for a weakening of this family duty.[2]

Japan has the world's longest life expectancy, which means that the oldest people are very old and, at the same time, often have children who are too old to be carers for them. According to the Ministry of Health and Welfare, in Japan half of the family carers in 1997 were over sixty. There is also a decreasing number of children. Thus, about half of the Japanese families have only one child. An explanation for this may be that an increasing number of Japanese women no longer seem to be attracted by the self-sacrificing family role and therefore delay marriage and childbirth (Auestad 2005). Furthermore, the unemployment rate in Japan is small (4.4% in 2005) compared with other countries in the Organisation for Economic Co-operation and Development, and about half of the labor-age women are in the labor market. In other words, although some people still might be willing to support their parents, the basis for realizing this willingness is reduced.

This general picture of Japanese family duty is very different from the Norwegian one and several of the demographic challenges in Japan are quite absent in Norway. As a matter of fact, there has been no tradition of several generations living together in Norway. An exception is the situation where, for example, a lone, unmarried woman might take care of a mother or father who is dependent on nursing. But the main Norwegian norm within this area has been that two women never share the same kitchen. Thus, there is a fundamental difference in family relationships between Japan and Norway, although it can be said that they are moving in the same direction. But it is too easy to say that these differences are merely about a displacement in time. Rather, we face two very different historical family traditions. And the central difference seems to be that in Norway family ties can be strong, even though part of the duty of support is handed over to the state. Historically, the root for this change can be found in the Social Care Act of 1964, which decreed that Norwegian children no longer had the formal duty to take care of their parents. Although this duty in praxis, to a certain degree, is independent of the law, this law signals that the formal demands of informal care for older family members are quite weak in Norway.

On the basis of the above mentioned differences in timing and history and as an introduction to the following analysis, we can contend that at the time when Norwegian elderly care is a challenging issue in the late modern phase, Japanese elderly care is starting on its first phase. However, as I point out in the following discussion, this first phase of Japanese elderly care includes more than merely traditional elements.

Traditional care

The first Norwegian phase saw the establishment of publicly organized home-based care. Some early Norwegian care studies describe the characteristics of this phase. These studies (Lie 1987; Ones 1988; Wærness 1982) show that relations between caregivers and care recipients were characterized by qualities such as closeness and consideration for the individual recipient. They also show a widespread gratitude among the elderly for receiving home care services. Because the services provided by the caregivers were based on a deep respect for the person as an unique person in need, and through combined rationality and empathy in the same act, the sociologist Kari Wærness (1984) found it timely to introduce a different and overlooked type of rationality in society. She called it a *rationality of caring* (see Chapter 1). Furthermore, there were few professional rules for the care work, and although the caregivers had no theoretical knowledge, they had considerable experience-based knowledge of care work in general and of housework from their own private homes. A striking feature of the organization of care work during this phase was that employees had few but regular clients. Together with the fact that there were few rules for the work, this meant that it was possible to develop a qualitative nearness to the individual elderly person.

The care researcher Marta Szebehely (1995) has identified three ways in which home care work was organized in Sweden. She calls the model that she constructs to account for the abovementioned characteristics a *traditional model*. Thus there existed structural organizational conditions for home help in this period, providing opportunities for the development of care-rational acts. The famous classical sociological idea about Gemeinschaft, a community based on qualitative nearness, was developed by Ferdinand Tönnies (1963) and seems to consist of similar characteristics, although Tönnies used the family as a typical example. The impact of doing this work in the privacy of the home, the possibility of closeness between carers and caregivers, and the weak control from outside seen together give rise to the tight bonds of those communities that Tönnies called Gemeinschaft. And, central to this care, Gemeinschaft is the possibility for rational acts, which can only proceed on the basis of respect for the person dependent on help and a certain degree of freedom in time and action for the caregiver to act naturally (immanent) without prescriptions and regulations (Christensen 1998b). Indeed, there were further structural conditions for care-rational acts during this phase.

From a legal point of view, home help work was covered by the Social Care Act, the same law that weakened the duties between children and parents. But in the practice of care-giving work, no attention was given to these legal aspects. Consequently, control and regulation of home help was weak and of marginal consideration.

With the possible exception of the social-political idea that elderly people should have the possibility of living in their own homes as long as possible, there was no dominant national ideology during this phase. This means there was little ideological significance in the work that was actually done during care work. The way this work was carried out therefore depended primarily on the value orientation of the individual employee. Studies of this phase show a general desire to develop personal relations with clients, and the presence of altruistic motives among caregivers (Lie 1987: 60; Wærness 1982: 146). This kind of value orientation can be understood in terms of the experience of care and housework that these caregivers had from their own homes.

It is crucial to mention that, especially during this early phase of modernization, the field of care giving was almost exclusively a woman's world. The majority of both employees and elderly recipients were women, and from a quantitative point of view this is still the case. But from a qualitative point of view, the position of the woman has changed since this early phase. The early phase was dominated by a traditional view of female responsibilities, with women being recruited from experienced housewives. There was no tradition of trade unions and no focus on the role of being an employee. In this light, the altruism mentioned above implies that home helpers sometimes did more for their clients than they were paid for (Wærness 1982: 145). In fact, it was this interesting aspect of home helpers' activity that formed the empirical foundation for the *rationality of caring* concept (Wærness 1996). Doing work without getting paid for it was an irrational action when judged by the values of the paid labor market. However, in the field of home-based care, this was meaningful and rational. This also explains the dilemma of these home helpers arising from the conflict between traditional feminine values derived from the family sphere and values derived from the labor market (Wærness 1982; Christensen 1998b).

In summing up this early phase of modernization in the field of home care, it is essential to mention that the legal and ideological control of the field was weak and unfocused. This meant that the women who performed this care work tended to let the informal values of family care determine the value orientation of their professional work, thereby contributing to what a sociologist might call Gemeinschaft in this field. Due to the lack of explicit and clear control, it was possible to foster the rationality of care within the sphere of care interactions. The indispensable condition for this situation was the presence of women with experiences of care work in the family, altruistic attitudes, and practical competence to act according to this pattern. But it would be wrong to suppose that home care during this phase was idyllic. The negative side of this picture is that the work was poorly paid, often consisting of very small part-time commitments. Furthermore, it was of low status, protected by very few workers' rights, and it was lonely work, since it consisted exclusively of activities performed within the homes of elderly people without any contact with other home help workers. As we shall see, these problematic aspects of the work improved, but together with a transition of the care Gemeinschaft. And this is exactly what Tönnies's theory is about—the transition from a traditional to a modern society reflecting a change from the strong ties of Gemeinschaft (community) to the weaker ties of Gesellschaft (association). Thus, this field is now facing the challenges of maintaining a rationality that will soon lose its conditions when the services undergo further modernization. But even when Norwegian home helpers had weak employment conditions, the first step was taken to improve these same conditions.

In this early phase the weak employment conditions of the home helpers was a dark side of the Norwegian Gemeinschaft. The Japanese case is different. Here it becomes obvious that the burden on the families, often daughters or daughters-in-law, is the dark side of (family) Gemeinschaft as long as the state takes no comprehensive responsibility for elderly care. In this comparative perspective three points will be mentioned about the Japanese system. First, in Japan the family duty ideology seems to hinder people from fully accepting help from strangers. Second, the 10% fee payable if public support is allocated can be expensive for low-income groups and can encourage them to reduce the need for help from the public government. And, third, it is worth mentioning that it is too early to talk about a corresponding first step of improved conditions for female care workers, although forces in Japan (such as the trade union Rengo, for example) are aiming at this (see Chapter 3). Thus, in Japan today female predominance, part-time work, low pay, low status, and unqualified work are challenges concerning care workers doing the face-to-face work in private homes, institutions, and so on.[3] Using the concept of Gemeinschaft again, we can say that while the Norwegian Gemeinschaft was found in the public sphere of home care services in the 1970s, this is the potential situation in Japan after the year 2000. But while the Norwegian case in its early phase has conditions strengthening Gemeinschaft, many aspects of the long-term insurance system are hindering this in Japan.

Modern services

If we look at the Norwegian field of home-based care as a form of activity slowly moving from an outside position to one increasingly integrated in the traditional paid labor market, we see that it closely reflects a more general social development. In a classical sociological theory developed by Max Weber (1994), the modern development of society following the industrial revolution was characterized as a general process of rationalization. Weber used this term to highlight the trend towards increased specialization, standardization, and formalization with the objective of achieving greater effectiveness, rationality, and stability. Thus, bureaucratization, which means increasing control and regulation, is a crucial part of rationalization. And professionalization is another crucial part of rationalization, pointing to the fact that work increasingly is based on education and theoretical reflections. Applying this analysis of modernization to the welfare state society, the objective becomes especially distinct when the welfare state reaches the limit at which increased use of the public sector no longer seems the best and only way to meet society's welfare requirements. In the field of home-based services, this development started to become clear in the 1980s. Thus, we find a *bureaucratization* of elderly care services and a *professionalization* of the caregivers.

Starting with the institutional framework, we can mention the kind of circumstances that strengthen bureaucratization. Whereas the organization of care work used to be based on the model of just a few regular clients for each home help, it is now based on the model of many rotating clients. Szebehely calls the latter 'the assembly line model' (Szebehely 1995). The aim of this development is to divide the work in the home into separate and clearly defined tasks that are allocated to an increasingly diverse group of care recipients. In addition, these recipients are getting services from an increasingly diverse group of service providers. This change towards separation and standardization in care work reflects broader trends in the industrial sector and is therefore sometimes referred to as *Taylorism*, named after Frederick Winslow Taylor (Eliasson 1992; Taylor 1916). This change is central to the transition from Gemeinschaft to Gesellschaft because the new way of organizing these services also changes the relationships between carers and caregivers. In other words, this weakens the ties and the care work becomes more regulated and controlled.

Ideologically, these changes were strengthened by a new ideology. Although the ideology that encouraged people to remain at home for as long as possible was strengthened in this second phase, it seems to coincide with the much clearer value orientation of the so-called ideology of rehabilitation (Christensen and Næss 1999). The official aim of the latter was to change the view of elderly people as weak and dependent and to see them as people with resources. In practice this ideology encourages people to care for themselves, yet many elderly people cannot manage this. Responsibility is therefore easily passed on to relatives and others who are close to elderly people and who might be able to provide informal care when the welfare state cannot do so. New requests for elderly people to be more independent with resources corresponded well with the new changes for effectiveness and clearly defined care services.

From a legal point of view, the 1980s was an important decade. A law passed in 1984 moved responsibility for public care from a higher administrative level to a lower, local level. This law, the Law on Nursing Services in Municipality, promoted decentralization and coordination. On a higher institutional level, this coordination meant that the municipality had to make it possible for both institutional and home-based care for elderly people to be managed on the same level. On a lower institutional level, the coordination implied an integration of home help and home nursing. The two types of coordination are called the *big integration* and the *small integration* (NOU 1986: 4). The main providers, according to these changes in law, were the welfare state/welfare municipalities and the local organizations and their representatives. In 1988 additions were made to the law of 1984, and entailed responsibility for nursing homes being passed to the Norwegian municipalities. This was a further step towards major integration between home-based care and institutional care.[4] In this context it is also important to mention that the idea of coordination coincided with a reduction in the number of days people stayed in hospital. Consequently, home-based care came under pressure to relieve the pressure on hospitals. In Japan this phenomenon is called *social hospitalization* and it is seen as one of the major reasons for introducing the long-term care system in 2000. However, in Japan this was not primarily caused by an attempt at strengthening home-based care. Rather, it was, for example, caused by the fact that there was often nobody to take care of elderly people in their own homes. Furthermore, old Japanese people tended to prefer hospitals to old age homes, which for this generation easily raise fear of being stigmatized as poor (Saito 2002).

In the Norwegian case, the professionalization of the services can be seen as a consequence of institutional changes due to higher claims on nursing care, local administration, professionally argued solutions, and so on. However, this process is also a consequence of changes in the identity of those who became employees. Professionalization is not just about more formal education. We have to understand it as a much wider concept that covers any change relating to the entire work situation, including how that work is understood. It is also important to note that professionalization is most distinct among those with least formal education, especially the home helpers. For this group, professionalization meant a change of identity from that of housewife to that of employee, whereby the latter was associated with wages, organized labor, and a move towards improved knowledge (Christensen 1998b; Lie 1987). But, of course, professionalization also involved more formal education. Among other things, the reduction in in-patient time in hospitals and in relief places for respite care at various health institutions, and the growing population of very old people, increased the need for nursing care for elderly people (Christensen and Næss 1999). Although the most acute need was for home nurses, there was also a need for home helpers. In Norway a new vocational training was established during this phase, which could be pursued either directly after secondary school, or following a certain period of practical experience in the field of care. This four-year training encompassed two years of theory and two years of practice (Høst 1997). The demand for professionalization arose from organizational and demographic changes, but it had a significant and direct impact on caregivers and their relations to care recipients. It should also be mentioned that raised levels of formal knowledge among employees helped to improve confidence in elderly care. Viewed in this way, professionalization of the care workers became a kind of solution to modern bureaucratization and increased efficiency.

For their part, recipients became more differentiated in terms of age, need for nursing, cultural identity, and lifestyle (Christensen and Næss 1999). In other words, whereas some of them were able to meet the modern demand on them not to be mere recipients, most of them were not. It is worth noting that the Norwegian terms for care recipients changed during the 1980s from *clients* and *patients* to *users*, and that this change of rhetoric signaled increasing resources among care recipients. If we view this in association with the ideology of rehabilitation, which became increasingly clear in this phase, the user concept implies the idea of giving more responsibility to the recipients themselves. The demographic changes that occurred during this phase, which resulted in increased numbers of very old, sick, and lonely people, meant that this idea of presumed increased resources among the recipients was a largely unrealistic project (Christensen and Næss 1999). Furthermore, there was a reduction in the numbers of daughters and daughters-in-law as carers because they were increasingly absorbed into the general labor market in the 1980s (Christensen and Næss 1999). In other words, in this phase an increasing discrepancy arose between the dominant ideology in elderly care and the reality of increasing dependence among old people. And here we have the crucial point of the modern phase: an increasing discrepancy between, on the one hand, bureaucratization, professionalization, and the ideology of rehabilitation, and, on the other hand, the situation and needs of the recipients, such as the need of many old people for regular helpers (Christensen 1998b; Næss and Wærness 1996; Rønning 1995) and the need among caregivers to be able to offer what was really needed (Næss and Wærness 1996: 37). Instead of developing the rich resources that existed in the traditional phase, the rationalization of the services ignored and destroyed it. In other words, the possibilities of strengthening a rationality of caring interactions between caregivers and care recipients were obviously reduced (Bungum 1994).

Summing up the Norwegian changes within its second phase, it fulfilled all the structural and ideological conditions for modern public care by bureaucratizing its services and professionalizing its care workers. But this also meant that a tension between the services provided and the actual care needs was established. The earlier tendency of Gemeinschaft had been replaced by a tendency of Gesellschaft. Although some isolated characteristics from this phase, like the hospitalization issue, can be compared to a corresponding issue in Japanese elderly care, it is the assumption in this chapter that there is no corresponding *phase* of modernization to be found in Japan. Rather, the Japanese system seems to combine a traditional foundation for a welfare system with several elements of late modern characteristics, as we will see in the following section.

Late modern outputs

At the end of the second Norwegian phase the modern model of bureaucracy was supplemented by a new model that focused on quite different issues. This new model was called *new public management* (Pedersen 2001; Vabø 2001) and began to affect the field of care in the 1990s. This model encompassed ideas from market economics, which have obvious influence in the field of care in relation to documentation of care services, quality control, and competition and user orientation. Among the many scientists analyzing late modernity, Zygmunt Bauman is one who has paid particular attention to the general impact of the private market (Bauman 2005). While the relation between the individual and society earlier was regulated by the working ethic, Bauman finds that this function now is replaced by consumerism. Individuals are no longer integrated into society through their employment but through their consumerism. Although Bauman perhaps broadens this view too much (Nilsen 2007), the key idea within this general theory reflects an important change within the late phase of Norwegian elderly care by pointing at the major influence on services of ideas and forces from the private market. And, particularly, we can draw our attention to the idea of the so-called individualized customer and the new conditions for acting in life. As it is supposed in these theories, the conditions are no longer stable, but fluent. The individual is now forced to make choices in all parts of life. This famous idea Bauman shares with several other central modernity thinkers and, in general, it is called *individualization*. However, Bauman does not interpret these new conditions as freedom, but rather as a new form of control and discipline. With these late modern ideas in mind, I will now point at changes in the field of care in order to persuade the reader of a late modern phase in this field and will discuss corresponding Japanese issues.

A central change, which resulted from the Social Services Act of 1991, was a new requirement for a formal legally based care plan every time a citizen receives a social service (Christensen 2001; Thorsen 1998). The consequence of this requisition is that municipal practice changed from being flexible and informal to rule-based and formal. The requisition specifies how much help the recipient will receive from the welfare state and for how long. Furthermore, this requisition supplies recipients with information about their right to complain. If they complain and are proved right, the amount of help given has to be revised and a new requisition is required. Also, each requisition has to be renewed when the time allocated has ended. In addition to the legal requisition, many Norwegian municipalities provide a formal agreement describing in detail which tasks will be performed by the recipient and which by the caregiver. Thus, by this new law, the relationship between the caregiver and the care receiver is changed into a relationship between two parties having a contract. And in this new contractual relationship, the care receiver has become a *consumer* and the care provider a *service deliverer*. This change is also strengthened by important structural changes in the way services are organized and allocated.

Regarding the organization, the model in this phase is dominated by what Szebehely has called a 'self-regulated small group model' (Szebehely 1995). This model is based on the assembly line model, with the difference that the caregivers and recipients are individualized. They have broader rights, but at the same time both parties are more replaceable and their interaction is greatly reduced. It is no longer important *who* is giving help to *whom*; the services rendered have become independent of both parties—and this amounts to a further step away from care rationality. There may well be a time lag in this late modern process of change among recipients, since there are still many old people who find it easier to show gratitude than to take the initiative to order the services they require from commercial providers. But most likely this will change when the rights-oriented generations replace the grateful generations. In Norway this would most likely include women and men born in the 1940s who were young in the 1960s, a radical period in Europe. In Japan these changes, rather than being about a shifting within the public sphere, include a shift from close family bonds to contractual public relations. With its new long-term care system, Japan has jumped the intermediate phase and has gone straight into new late modern orientations.

Another change strengthening the new consumer-service delivery relation in Norway concerns the process of help allocation. While previously the caregiver and care recipient made an informal agreement about the details of the help to be supplied, the new procedure involves a formal clarification of the recipient's specific needs (Vabø 2001). This model, called a *purchaser–provider model*, results in formalization and standardization of the work of assigning services. The principal feature of the model is that assignment of the kind and amount of work to be performed in the individual household is made by employees who do not, themselves, perform those services. We are here dealing with a new separation of care planning on the one hand and the performance of the care work on the other. But while this introduces a change from a more informal system in the Norwegian system, this has been a characteristic of the Japanese long-term care system from its beginning. Within this system people are assessed by answering eighty-two standard questions about their daily needs. The answers are analyzed by a computer system, and a group of professionals (nurses, doctors, social workers, etc.)

makes a decision about the final amount of support (worth a certain amount of yen) to allocate (Saito 2002). Afterwards, the user can choose the care service (for example, to go to a day service center) and the service provider, which can be a private company, a cooperative, an association, and so on. Then the services follow a contract and this also implies that the user can complain about the quality of the services.

It is obvious that this is a model introducing a very controlled and standardized system for public elderly care in Japan. Two central questions following this model are whether the computer-based system actually manages to evaluate needs in a fair manner and whether the quality of services can be controlled when it is provided by profit-based organizations. Actually, it is interesting that the number of private companies, in the beginning, did not increase as much as expected because the care compensations seemed to be too low to make these companies profitable (Saito 2002: 210). Now, the numbers seem to have increased, particularly in the biggest cities (see Chapter 6).

The Norwegian process of allocating support seems to be less standardized, although standardization has increased, together with the separation of the care planning and the performance of the tasks. In addition, local (e.g. Gerix), as well as national (e.g. IPLOS), standard measure systems have been developed in order to produce statistical overviews of needs and to use them for working out general care plans. Thus, it is likely that the difference between the Norwegian and the Japanese case mostly lies in how much this is used in the process of assessing people's needs. Also, the idea of letting the users choose their services and service providers has a Norwegian parallel.

In Norway's late phase the field of care has become open to a policy of privatizing services. This development began in the modern phase but became much more explicit in the late modern phase. There are several types of privatization, but the most tested one is open competition, where the welfare municipality competes with private agents in offering services on the open market. This tendency became even clearer in the 2000s, when another contribution to privatization was added to public services through a model called 'user's free choice' (St.meld.nr.25 2005–06). This means that when the local authority has allocated a certain amount of help to a person, this person has the option to choose between caregivers employed by the municipality or caregivers employed by a private company contracted by the municipality. Although this model is not yet very widespread across Norway, it signals future developments, with users having more influence on services and the services provided. Internationally, some scientists call this phenomenon *empowerment* (see Askheim 2003). However, this raises the issue of how much empowerment is actually realized when people do not have the resources necessary to make real choices, when the degree of choice depends on local contexts, and when the services provided do not necessarily fit the needs, just to mention a few issues. Furthermore, in Norway research on the consequences of privatization indicates that employees experience insecurity about their working conditions in these new organizations (Bogen and Nyen 1998; Bogen 2001). An explanation for this is that in principle the organizations are oriented towards economic profit and are therefore likely to set aside other concerns that may incur expenses. Compared to the modern Norwegian phase, this insecurity concerning working conditions is an important factor in the current context when we consider that one aim in professionalizing the care sector was to strengthen the position and autonomy of employees (Christensen 1998a). In other words, privatization, whether practiced in Japan or in Norway, tends in the long run to weaken the role of the employee and hence risks weakening the position of women in the labor market.

To sum up, it is obvious that Japan has included several late modern values in its new insurance system in spite of its very traditional starting point based on a strong ideology of family duty. Bauman's ideas about consumerism and individualization are distinct in the Norwegian, as well as the Japanese, elderly care system and clarify that the relationship between the caregiver and the care recipient is now individualized within a context of standardized need assessments and allocations of support.

Challenges of modernizing care

In this chapter I have applied a perspective of modernization in order to analyze the development of elderly care in Norway critically. With this as my starting point, I have discussed differences, as well as similarities, between crucial Norwegian and Japanese solutions to public elderly care. The discussion is structured on the basis of three phases of modernity: a traditional, a modern, and a late modern phase. A central conclusion from this analysis is that despite the fact that Japan started its process of modernization at a time when Norway had fully entered its late modern phase, the two countries today seem to share several late modern values. However, this does not necessarily mean that they also share all the same challenges.

On the basis of general theory about welfare state regimes (Esping-Andersen 1990, 1999), a rosy picture of Norway easily arises in comparison with Japan, since the first is usually characterized as a social democratic state and the latter as a conservative welfare state. In this chapter I have questioned this rosy picture of Norwegian elderly care by pointing in particular to two main issues. First, it is obvious that in spite of the development of a care rationality due to Gemeinschaft conditions in Norway's early phase, the structural conditions for this were weakened more and more during the modern and late modern phases. Second, a major tension was established during the modern and late modern phases between the political ideas and solutions on the one hand and the actual needs of older people on the other. According to the historical key issues of modernity, Norwegian elderly care has undergone a revolution but it has failed to develop liberty for the care workers and older people with needs for care in everyday life. Norway shares late modern challenges related to individualization and consumerism with Japan. But, in addition, Japan faces a major challenge in the strong influence of a family ideology, which, first, blocks the development of a welfare state with comprehensive responsibility for its oldest citizens and, second, blocks female liberation from the heavy burdens of family commitments.

In the late modern phase the care services in Norway, as well as in Japan, adopted the notion of outputs by adapting ideas and models from the private market. This perspective allows them to see their activities from a commodity-producing perspective. But if the general future aim is to strengthen care rationality within this field, this kind of commodity-like productivity must be replaced by a new understanding of care. Care should not be reduced to limited standardized outputs, to commodities delivered at the door. It should be placed as one of the basic aspects of developing communities in society because of the fact that it can strengthen solidarity among citizens and make a significant contribution to the social inclusion of people depending on public help.

Chapter 3
Development of Home Help in Japan: A Comparison with Norway

Yayoi Saito

(Translated by Beverley Anne Yamamoto)

Introduction

Compared to the other Scandinavian countries, the Norwegian home help system was developed slightly later than in Denmark and Sweden. The home help system in Norway was institutionalized by the state in 1969, which is later than in Japan. Home help services were organized by voluntary organizations or municipalities in Norway before being institutionalization by the state.

The gap between home help provision widened and the configuration of the welfare state came to be totally different between 1970 and 1990. While Norway succeeded in achieving a well-organized home help system in this period, Japan did not. What factors contributed to these situations? On the other hand, in recent years there has been a tendency for long-term care services in the two countries to become similar in certain respects.

The aim of this chapter is to draw on Christensen's concept of the modernization of home help and Wærness's concept of the rationality of care to make comparisons between the development processes in Japan and Norway in order to clarify differences and similarities.

Drawing on a concept of bureaucracy and Wærness's *rationality of caring*, Christensen (2004: 35–6) divided the development process of home help services in Norway into three periods—*traditional care*, *modernization*, and *late modern outputs*. The first period, from the end of the Second World War until 1970, was before the bureaucratization of home help. After the end of the Second World War, Norway saw the rapid development of the welfare state, yet in 1950 home help services were organized as volunteer work by women's groups in Oslo (Christensen 2004: 36). The government first started to provide funding for home help services in 1969. With the help of this funding, the home help system expanded to cover the whole country. Wærness emphasizes that home help services had been organized voluntarily for seventeen years before they were institutionalized by the state (Wærness 2008: 364–5).

In the second period, in the 1980s, in order to legislate for reduced services, a number of principles were hammered out. According to Christensen (2004: 37), the 1980s were extremely important in the development of home help services in Norway from the point of view of the organizational framework. Legislation that came into effect in 1984 devolved responsibility for care to the municipalities, which had to bear the burden of providing both residential homes for the elderly and in-home care. Then in 1988, as a result of a revision of the law, authority over nursing homes was also passed to the municipalities. This decentralization of care services occurred at the same time that hospitals were requested to reduce the number of days that geriatric patients were admitted as in-patients (Christensen 2004: 39).

During this stage the identity of the home helper also underwent a change from the housewife in the home to a worker who received a wage, was organized, and worked to improve her/his knowledge (Christensen 2004: 40). In addition, society began to need both community nurses and home helpers, and new forms of occupational training began. The improvement of the education and training of home helpers brought about a heightened trust in elderly care and the professionalization of home helpers was a solution to the bureaucratism of the period (Christensen 2004: 40–1).

The third period was one of realization that the welfare state could no longer fulfill the responsibilities that had been placed on it in the 1970s. In other words, this was a period when the route of placing some responsibility for care back with individuals and families was hammered out.

According to Christensen, there was a major reform of in-home care provision in 1991 with the revision of the Social Services Law. With an exchange of contract required between carer and user, home help became formalized and rooted in regulations. Seen from a legal view point, this was initiated in order to strengthen the authority of both carer and user. However, it resulted in the authority of both being curtailed, as the needs of the user were not fulfilled and there was little prospect for the carer to provide an individualized service (Christensen 2004: 41–2).

What Christensen points to here is the paradox of care. There is the central desire for the care worker to keep her/his own individual identity, yet the move has been to formalize and standardize care services. In particular, the task of formalizing and standardizing services undermines the possibility of developing a 'rationality of caring' (Christensen 2004: 42–3).

There is a wealth of pioneering research on the development of home help services in the Japanese context. Earlier work took as key moments in this history the 1969 provision for 'dispatch of home help services' that targeted bedridden elderly on low incomes and the 1982 expansion of provision to cover bedridden elderly living in ordinary families (Kitaba 2001: 214). In addition, earlier research highlighted the ways in which home help for the elderly shifted as a result of changes in the welfare system and policy (Kitaba 2001: 214). Drawing on previous research, Kitaba (2001) set about clarifying the reasons for the change in the system of home help services for the elderly. In this chapter I will build on Kibata's work.

In addition, Christensen's (2004) concepts of traditional care, modernization, and late modern outputs are reflected in the analysis and organization of this chapter. Discussion of the development of home help services in Japan will be organized around Christensen's three periods. Figure 3.1 shows the increase in home helpers from 1962 to 2007. The number of home helpers was 250 in 1962, but it increased to 282,812 in 2007. It is difficult to divide the home help development period in Japan neatly into the three Christensen's phases because Japanese society experienced rapid aging during this period and Japanese policies had to catch up and adapt to such conditions. It seems that some phenomenon and reforms happened all at one time in Japan compared with Norway. But form of development is similar for both countries.

For the traditional care phase, I will focus on the period starting with the 1962 institutionalization of home help services for the elderly and follow through to the creation of the Ten-Year Strategy to Promote Health Care and Welfare for the Aged (Gold Plan) in 1989. Earlier research will be highlighted in order to underscore the reasons for the changes that took place in home help during this period.

During the second period of modernization, I will focus on the ten-year period in which the Gold Plan was being implemented—1990 through to 2000. During this period home help was increasingly organized and, under the Gold Plan, we saw the development of infrastructure throughout the country as services came to be provided at municipal level. The third period, that of late modern outputs, is defined as the period since the Long-Term Care Insurance (LTCI) System was introduced in 2000. Over the past nine years home help in Japan has been greatly influenced by the new public management model. Initially, the volume of home help expanded and the quality of the service provided changed greatly, but more recently (with the introduction of a concept of prevention) we have seen the start of cutbacks in services. Here I will compare the development of the home help system in Japan with that in the Scandinavian countries, with a special focus on a comparison with Norway. The special characteristics of the Japanese system will be elaborated and an analysis of the reasons for these will be undertaken.

Figure 3-1: Trends in the number of home helpers in Japan (1962–2007)

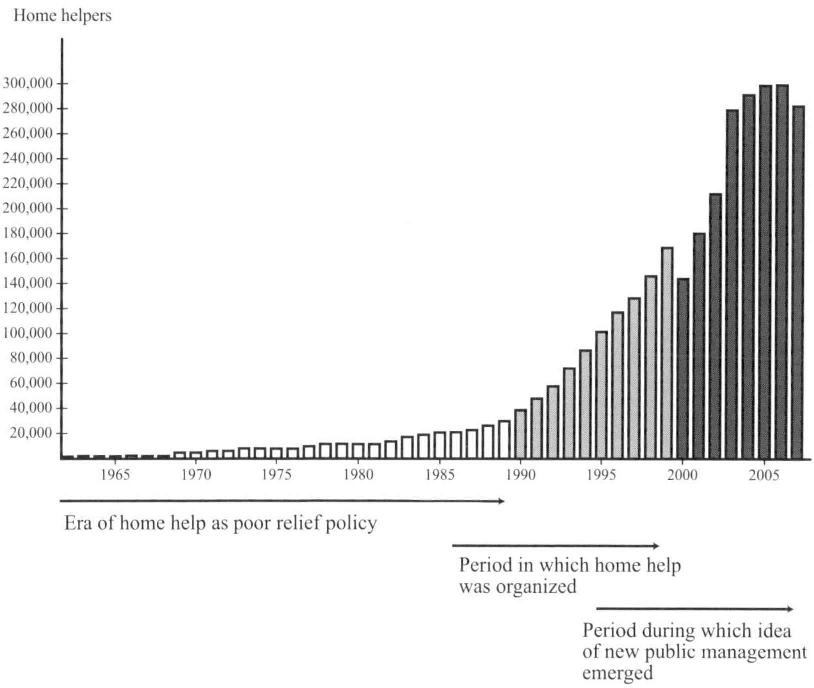

Note: The method of counting home helpers has changed since 2000.

Source: Based on Mori 1974, Kitaba 2001: 237, and the Ministry of Health, Labour, and Welfare (Japan)

The beginnings of home help and a poor relief policy (1962–89)

Home help as poor relief policy

It is somewhat surprising to find that the institutionalization of home help services by the state occurred earlier in Japan than in Norway. Compared to Norway, it started differently in Japan, where there was little expectation that home help would be provided on a voluntary basis.[1] From a legal angle, the system of home helpers for the elderly began in 1962,[2] when the dispatching of home helpers[3] formally became the responsibility of the state. However, the number dispatched was extremely small, at only 250 for the country; even then, they were only assigned in six cities, including Tokyo (Takaki 2006: 21).

In 1963 the Law for the Welfare of the Elderly (*Rōjin fukushi hō*) came into effect and made provisions for 'the municipality through social welfare corporations (*shakai fukushi hōjin*)[4] and other organizations to dispatch home helpers to the homes of elderly persons who were experiencing difficulty with daily living, whether due to physical or mental disability, to offer them support' (Article 12). As a result, home help services came to be legally deemed as one variety of social services. However, following on from this, this style of Japanese home helper (*rōjin katei hōshiin,* literally 'home servants for the elderly') hardly increased in number.

Figure 3.2 offers a comparison of the number of home helpers in three countries belonging to the International Council of Home Help Services (Mori 1974: 44). As also noted by Christensen (2004), from the 1970s the number of home helpers increased dramatically in Norway. Norway was in the group that has the highest number of home helpers of all member countries. As there is no breakdown by full- or part-time work status for Japan, it is not possible to make a full comparison. The number of home helpers in Japan increased little compared to Norway and Sweden during this period.

Table 3.1 shows the number of home helpers per 100 000 people. In 1973, compared to 825 in Sweden and 577 in Norway, in Japan there were just nine home helpers per 100,000 people. Thus, even though there was a home help system in Japan, the numbers involved were extremely low.

At the initial stage in Japan, the government had two purposes in introducing home help. One was to help the elderly who lived alone without family, and the other was to give jobs to widows and women who needed social assistance. As mentioned, the number of home helpers did not increase until the end of the 1980s.

Home help in the early period in Japan was strongly associated with the poor relief policy and only low-income elderly were targeted for this service. There were four reasons for this: (1) government policy was 'the Japanese-style social welfare model,' (2) the high rate of co-residence with other family members and the low aging rate, (3) the availability of cheap housekeepers, and (4) the stigma of taking social services.

The four reasons for late development of home help

The Japanese-style social welfare model

Compared to European countries, the amount spent on social security, expressed as a percentage of gross domestic product (GDP), is extremely low in Japan. Even in the period 1955 to 1975, when the country was experiencing rapid economic growth, Japanese social security expenditure was maintained at the low level of 2% of GDP. On this point, it can be said that the policy of the Japanese government concerning the direction of social welfare had

Figure 3-2: Trends in the number of home helpers (Norway, Sweden, and Japan)

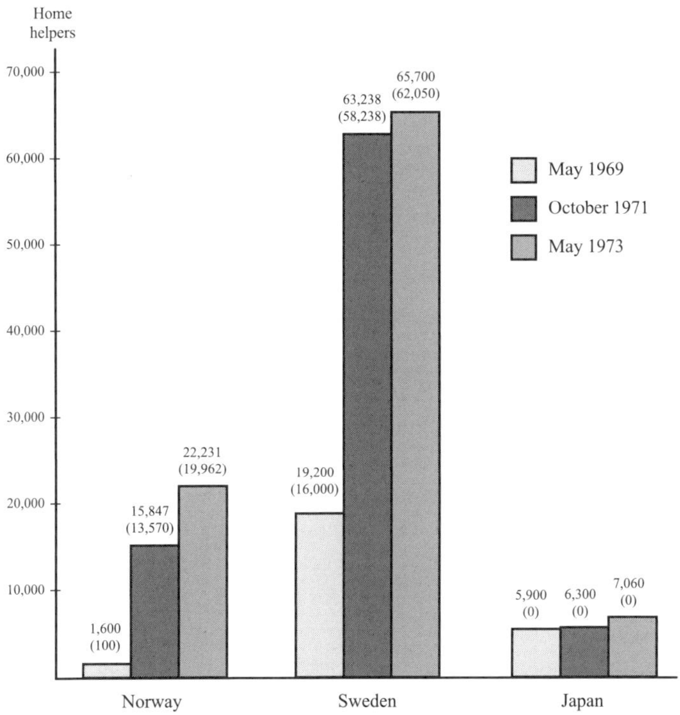

Note: The figures in brackets represent the number of part-time workers

Source: Based on Mori 1974: 7, 42. (Original source: The 1969 statistics come from the third General Assembly of the International Council of Home Help Services in Brussels, Belgium. The 1971 statistics come from the first International Seminar of the International Council of Home Help Services in Woudschoten, The Netherlands. The 1973 statistics come from the fourth General Assembly of the International Council of Home Help Services in London, United Kingdom.)

Table 3.1: The number of home helpers per 100 000 people

Country	October 1971	May 1973
Sweden	800	825
Norway	400	577
Japan	8	9

Source: Based on Mori 1974: 47. (Original source: the 1971 statistics come from the first International Seminar of the International Council of Home Help Services in Woudschoten, The Netherlands. The 1973 statistics come from the fourth General Assembly of the International Council of Home Help Services in London, United Kingdom.)

not undergone a massive change since the pre-war period (Goodman and Ito 1996: 201).

Goodman and Ito (1996) emphasize that since the mid-1970s Japan's social welfare system has diverged from the model of Western countries. This is called 'the Japanese-style social welfare model' (*Nihongata fuskushi shakai*) and is constituted with social security at the center and with a heavy dependency on the family to bear the burden of social welfare (Goodman and Ito 1996: 193).

Since its founding in 1955, the Liberal Democratic Party enjoyed a majority as the ruling party until 1967, when for the first time it lost its majority. As a result of losing its majority, the government raised pension benefits, instituted a system of free medical care for the elderly, and launched a policy of strengthening welfare policy to appease the voter (Goodman and Ito 1996: 203).

Nevertheless, with the 1974 oil shock acting as the trigger, there was a neo-conservative backlash against welfare state policies (Goodman and Ito 1996: 203). There was an about face on the line of policy to improve welfare provision that had been initiated less than ten years earlier. For example, the welfare systems of the United Kingdom and the Scandinavian countries became targets of criticism. It was suggested that if the welfare system was strengthened, it would not only cost a lot in terms of tax revenue, but would also cause a stagnation of the economy and Japan would suffer the 'British disease.' Others suggested that there had been an increase in suicide among the elderly because of welfare policy that had 'gone too far' and weakened the family. This kind of criticism was frequently expressed.

In this way, the Japanese welfare system through to the 1980s held on to the conservative undercurrent from the pre-war period, but, in reaction to economic conditions, welcomed the functions of the welfare state on a small scale. The reasons why social security on a small scale became possible were that the rate of co-residence with family was high and companies had instituted their own independent welfare programs such as accommodation allowances and health management (Goodman and Ito 1996: 201).

The assumption that lay behind the Japanese-style social welfare model was that men would earn the family wage and women would care for their families. In other words, it is premised on the so-called *bread-winner model* of gender relations. Figure 3.3 shows trends in the female labor force participation rate from 1972 to 2005 for Sweden, Norway, and Japan. In 1972 the female labor force participation rate in Norway was 44.7% and it was slightly lower than in Japan at 47.7%. But significant differences emerged between Norway and Japan in the 1970s and 1980s, as more and more women entered the workforce in Norway, while the same did not occur in Japan. The Japanese

Figure 3-3: Trends in the female labor force participation rate, 1972–2005 (Sweden, Norway, and Japan)

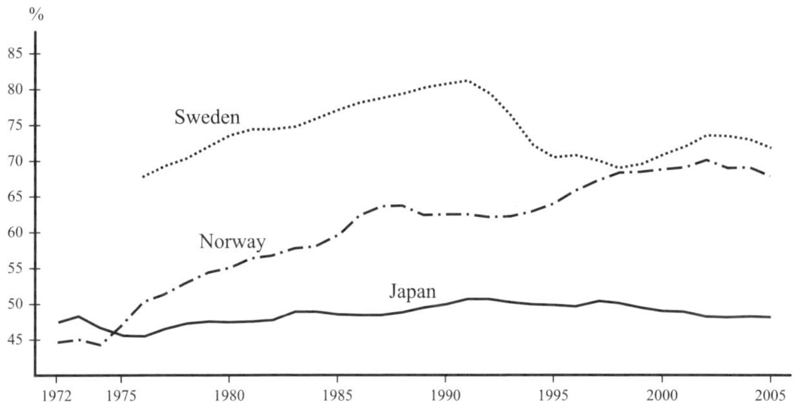

Source: Sweden, Statistiska centralbyrån; Norway, Statistisk sentralbyrå; Japan, Statistics Bureau, Ministry of Internal Affairs and Communications

government revised its tax policy and pension scheme during this period to reward housewives to stay at home.

The high rate of co-residence

During the 1970s and 1980s a high percentage of elderly were co-residing with their adult children. In 1970, 73.4% of elderly were living with their children, and, despite a decrease, in 1985 the figure was still 64.6% (see Figure 3.4). The concomitant increase in the number of elderly living alone was not raised as a social problem at this time. The custom of the oldest son staying on in the maternal home continued. Even if there was a temporary separation, it was common once an elderly parent was in need of care that she or he would co-reside with the eldest son and his family. Furthermore, for families with a certain degree of affluence, there were cases where the parent and child co-resided and outside housekeeping services were purchased.

In addition, if we look at population dynamics, compared to many European countries where there was an urgent response to the aging of society, in Japan the rate of elderly in the population was still low (Figure 3.5). In 1975 the population aging rate was extremely low in Japan at 7.9%, compared to 13.7% in Norway and 15.1% in Sweden. There were very few home help workers and they were only dispatched to the homes of elderly living alone on low incomes, but this did not prompt much debate.

Figure 3-4: Percentage of elderly aged sixty-five and over co-residing with their children (Japan)

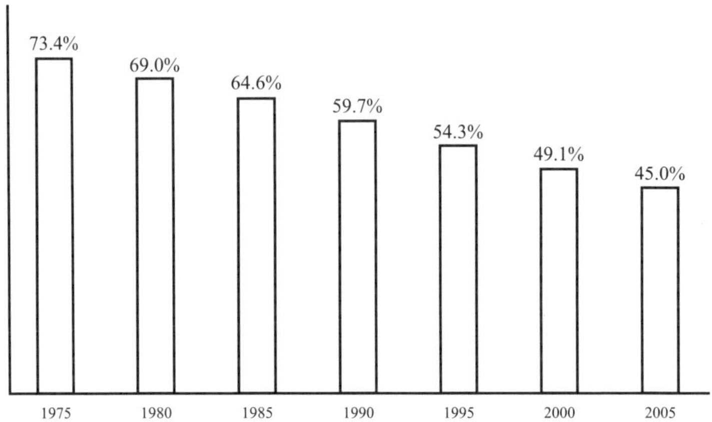

Source: Ministry of Health, Labour, and Welfare (Japan) 2007

The pre-war family system exerted a significant influence on attitudes to home help services. Even in the post-war period, the idea was deeply entrenched that caring for family members was something that should be undertaken by the family at home. In the pre-war Japanese Civil Code, children were charged with a duty to support their parents. In return for being the successor of the household, the oldest son was obliged to live with his parents and to care for them until they died. Should a parent become ill and be in need of nursing or care, the eldest son's wife was expected to take on this role. In addition, the Imperial Rescript on Education (*Kyōiku ni kansuru Chokugo*)[5] gave young people during the pre-war period a thorough education in the ethos of filial piety.

The Poor Relief Law (*Kyūgo hō*) that came into effect in 1901 was applied to those elderly without relatives to look after them, and Homes of the Elderly Poor (*yōrō-in*) were provided for this group. These homes were inferior environments and not desirable conditions in which to live daily life.

The old Civil Code was abolished after the end of the Second World War, and Article 25 of the new Constitution states that 'All people shall have the right to maintain minimum standards of wholesome and cultured living' and to enjoy social rights. It was as a result of Article 25 of the new Constitution that the basis of a social security system was created in roughly the first decade of the post-war period. However, the image of social services being a part of poor relief policy remains strong, especially among those educated

Figure 3-5: Trends in the population aging rate (Norway, Sweden, and Japan)

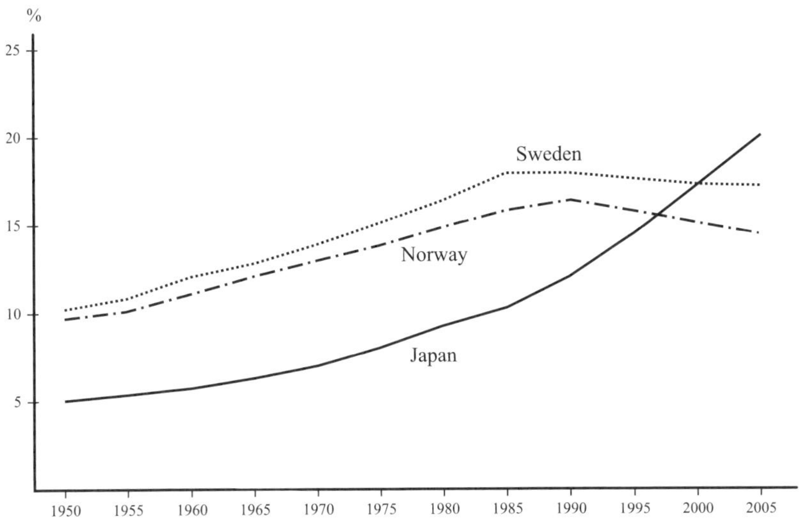

Source: Based on Population Division of the Department of Economic and Social Affairs of the United Nations (2009).

in the pre-war period. It is also important that home help in Japan was only offered to elderly on low incomes and took as its departure point the characteristic of being poor relief (Mori 1974: 17).

Competition with paid housekeepers and housewives

The third explanation for home help being offered as poor relief is the existence of paid domestic help. Paid domestic helpers received relatively low wages and, along with the housewife, who engaged in unpaid care work, they were competition for home helpers. Figure 3.6 shows trends in the number of domestic workers in Japan.

In the early post-war period it was usual not only for upper-class families but also middle-class families to have housemaids (*jyotyū*). There were housemaids in the pre-war period also, which provided not only a place for young women to work, but also somewhere that manners could be learned prior to marriage. In many cases, young women from rural areas were particularly likely to become housemaids (Kitaba 2001: 223).

From the beginning of the twentieth century, opportunities for women to work in factories increased and the number of young women willing to live-in and work as housemaids declined accordingly. However, there was an

Figure 3-6: Trends in the number of domestic workers in Japan

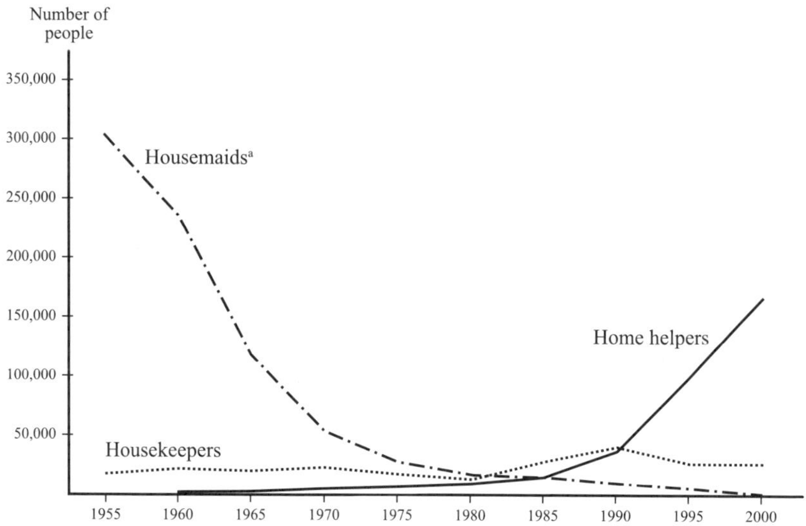

Note: a = Housemaids means live-in housekeepers here.

Source: Based on Kitaba 2001: 224. Ministry of Health, Labour, and Welfare (Japan) and Ministry of Internal Affairs and Communications (Japan)

increase in housekeepers (*kaseifu*) who lived out. In 1927 there were 510,000 housekeepers and housemaids throughout Japan (Kitaba 2001: 223).

After the mid-1960s Japan experienced a period of rapid economic growth, which demanded a massive labor force within the country and, as a consequence, maids' work came to be shunned (Kitaba 2001: 223). In the pre-war period, if a family member was ill, not only would a doctor be asked to make a home visit but a home nurse would be hired to care for the patient until he or she recovered (Kitaba 2001: 223).

Despite a rise in the number of home helpers since 1980, the number of housekeepers did not decline. One reason is thought to be that housekeepers were hired to accompany the elderly who were admitted to hospital. Housekeepers who chaperoned the elderly to hospital in order to look after their needs slept by the sick bed and were called 'chaperone women' (*tsukisoifu*) and could be seen until very recently. In principle, the practice of having *tsukisoifu* in hospitals was abolished in 1996, yet cases are still seen today of a person being hired by the family to accompany an elderly person with senile dementia while in hospital. According to Mori (1974), one of the reasons that the institutionalization of home helpers initially did not extend to the ordinary household was the vested interests of private enterprises offering housekeeping services (Mori 1974: 17).

Resistance to outsourcing care

Akeyama and Nogawa (1975) carried out a survey of municipalities that had implemented the home helper (home service) for elderly homes system. From this it was found that many respondents expressed the opinion that to expand home help services would weaken family relationships. The following types of comments were made:

> An upgrading [of the service] for elderly living alone is needed, but seen from the viewpoint of family relationships there might be a negative effect with bedridden elderly.
>
> As a result of dispatching home service workers a situation may arise where the family become more distant and there will be many households who subsequently leave things undone for many days. Before we start debating the merits of expanding the system, the priority should be to strengthen the family's duty to care (Akeyama and Nogawa 1975: 346–7).

Upon receiving the results of the survey, Akeyama and Nogawa advised that while a certain level of service could be provided to relieve some of the fatigue of the family, the objective was to have the family do the caring and to provide some assistance. They argued that providing too much in the way of services would genuinely undermine the welfare of the elderly person (Akeyama and Nogawa 1975).

Similarly, in the 1962 Ministry of Health and Welfare White Paper (*Kōsei Hakusho*) it was stated that 'the task of [the] home service worker project was not an easy one...as the name suggests it literally requires a spirit of service' (*hōshiteki na kimochi*) (Sasaki 2005: 8), showing that the government's position was that the work of the home helper required a sense of service.

In past research it has also been theorized that as a result of the state institutionalizing home help services, they were introduced in Japan selectively as a character of poor relief. However, the reason for this was that in order to make it a national system, it was necessary to emphasize the poor relief aspect. An international comparison suggests that the strong bureaucratism in Japan that had existed from the pre-war period acted as a barrier to the birth of altruistic volunteerism or feminism.

The period during which home help was organized (1990s)

The organization of home help in Japan

Home help as general service

Looking back at Figure 4.1, the increase in the number of home helpers after 1982 displayed a slightly different pattern. This reflects the revision of the system that took place in 1982.

The revision of the system[6] with the introduction of the Management Outline of Home Helpers (*Rōjin Katei Hōshiinn jigyō unei yōkō*) made it possible to dispatch, for a fee, home helpers even to homes that were not low income (Article 7). In addition, the work of the home helper that had previously been recognized only as full-time work was now made available on a part-time basis (Article 8). According to the revision, home helpers were requested to be physically and mentally healthy, to have passion for and understanding of elderly care, and to have ability and experience in housekeeping, elderly care, and advising (Article 8).

While it brought in a payment-for-services regime, in a sense the reform freed home help services from the link with the poor relief policy, as users were no longer limited to low-income households. Early Japanese research points to 1982 as a turning point in the history of home help in Japan (Suga 2001; Kitaba 2001).

However, the problem was the absolute shortage of service capacity. While from a systems level an elderly person was entitled to make use of home help services, in reality very few could. Even in 1982 there were fewer than forty home helpers for every 1000 bedridden elderly living at home (The Tenth Quality-of-life Policy Council 1986). As a result, elderly living alone were given priority and those co-residing with family continued to be forced to provide all care themselves, and thus there was no change.

If we compare this with Norway and Sweden, from the 1980s onwards Japan finally started to provide a home help service for households that were not low income. From the mid-1980s the need for some kind of help from neighbors was discussed and volunteer activities centering mainly on housewives began to appear. Although the number of official home helpers did not increase, with the advancement of the aging of society it became impossible to bear the burden of care just within the family.

It is interesting that two nationwide organizations were appeared as civil movement in this period. In 1980 the Alzheimer's Association of Japan[7] was established in Kyoto. In the field of elderly welfare this was the first support group involving those caring for an elderly person to work at a national level. These people, who had experiences of caring for family members with dementia, called for an improvement in services.

In 1983 the Women's Association for the Better Aging Society[8] was formed in Tokyo and its group activities came to be conducted on a national level. In this movement there was a coming together of feminist activism and activism aimed at improving elderly care services. These two groups of activists became the driving force behind the implementation of the Gold Plan and the LTCI System, which will be discussed later.

Feminist and housewife groups active around issues of elderly care began as small local endeavors, but later became nationwide organizations and revealed a new wave of civil organization. While members of these groups did not work as voluntary caregivers, they were quite active in studying and discussing elderly care issues. Furthermore, they sometimes worked politically together as a lobbying group. Women who had experienced care for the elderly at home comprised the majority of group members. We can say that the elderly care issue had become a general issue for all people in the 1980s because the number of frail elderly had increased so rapidly, and, as a result, people were not able to cope with the heavy burden of family-based care.

The Gold Plan and the municipal elderly care plans

At the time that the Ministry of Health and Welfare[9] launched its Ten-Year Strategy to Promote Health Care and Welfare for the Aged (Gold Plan) in 1989, the government planned to increase the approximately 30,000 home helpers to 100,000 by the year 2000.

The Gold Plan set about developing the infrastructure for elderly care and for the first time in Japan set numerical targets. All 3200 municipalities at the time were required to carry out a lifestyle fact-finding survey of the care needs of elderly living within their municipalities. On the basis of the results, the need for care services through to the year 2000 was calculated and welfare plans for the elderly for each municipality were drawn up. In 1989 the Japanese name of workers carrying out care in the home was changed from 'home servants for the elderly' (*rōjin katei hōshiin*) to 'home helpers' (*hōmu herupa-*). As a result of the Gold Plan, 99.8% of municipalities had implemented a home help system by 1994.

The municipal elderly care plans,[10] which were published by all municipalities in Japan, suggested that many more than the initial Gold Plan target of 100,000 home helpers would be needed, with the results of the survey suggesting that at the very least 200,000 home helpers would be needed by

Table 3.2: Number of home helpers per population, Sweden, Norway, and Japan

	Number of home helpers	Per 100 000 people
Sweden (1985)	73,808	883.9
Norway (1983)	40,598	983.2
Japan (1985)	20,128	16.7

Source: Ogasawara 1991: 126.

the year 2000. In 1994 the government announced its New Gold Plan in which the target for home helpers by 2000 had been revised upwards to 170,000.

Table 3.2 shows the number of home helpers in relation to the population; however, Ogasawara's (1991) international comparison indicates how extremely low these were for Japan. Even after the fulfillment of the Gold Plan in 2000, Japan was not in the same league as the Scandinavian countries. Assuming that a twenty-four-hour system of home help was introduced, it was calculated that 600,000 home helpers—six times the number set as a target in the Gold Plan—would be needed (Ogasawara 1991: 125–6).

Occupational status of home helpers

Professionalization

In 1982 the qualifications of social worker and care worker were given legal recognition. It was legally stipulated that a social worker 'is a person with specialist knowledge and skills who is able to offer counseling, advice, and support to those with physical or mental disabilities, as well as those who are able to carry on with their daily life but due to environmental reasons are experiencing difficulties' (The Law of Social Workers and Care Workers (*Shakaifukushishi oyobi kaigo fukushishi hō*)). A social worker should basically have received four years of university education and is assumed to have counseling experience in a welfare facility.

It is stipulated that a certified care worker 'is a person with specialist knowledge and skills who engages in care work such as bathing, aiding bowel elimination, and meal preparation for a person who due to physical or mental disability has difficulty carrying out daily life activities, while also offering guidance on care to the person or their carers.' A care worker is someone who, after graduating from high school, has received two years of professional education at a technical college to gain certification and it is assumed that the care worker will provide services inside care institutions, as well as in-home services. Nevertheless, as the overwhelming majority of care workers would like to work in a welfare facility, there are not many certified who are willing to work as home helpers. Working in welfare facilities is more stable than home help.

In terms of hours of education for home helpers, in 1982 a total of seventy hours of training was introduced at the time of being hired, but this had been extended to 360 hours by 1987. In addition, the home servants of the elderly, who made up the entire body of home helpers, included, in part, widows who had been hired for employment by municipalities. The work of home helpers tended to be viewed as an extension of the job of the housewife and their professionalization came later than that of care workers in institutional facilities, and lower hurdles were set for them. Despite this, in 1994, fifty hours of training were necessary to receive the third-level home helper qualification, and 130 hours were necessary for level two. To receive home helper certification for level one, an additional 230 hours were needed. Thus, the movement to increase the professional education of home helpers was heightened.

Increase in the register model of home helpers

At the same time as home help was professionalized, the employment pattern changed. As mentioned above, in the early days it had been usual for home helpers (home servants for the elderly) to be municipal workers. Since the Gold Plan, however, there has been a decrease in home helpers employed directly by the municipality. Many municipalities came to contract out home help services to private organizations such as social welfare corporations.[11] The reason given for this trend is that it costs the municipality roughly twice as much in labor costs if it hires home helpers directly compared to hiring their services from a private organization. In addition, there are strict regulations concerning the working conditions of the former under the Local Public Service Law (*Chihō komuin hō*), which makes it impossible to hire in a flexible way.

Commissioning home help services from the private sector and the accompanying reduction in full-time work saw the popularization of a new register model of home helpers in the form of 'registered helpers' (*tōroku herupa-*). The registered helper registers the days that she or he would like to work and aims to only work on those days. However, if there is no work on that day, the helper gets no income. The registered helper has become the typical pattern of employment for home helpers throughout Japan. While this has brought about an increase in choice, in reality the work of the home helper has become unstable.

While the professionalization of home helpers was advanced through education, the introduction of the register model made it more difficult for home helpers to be economically independent in their work.

A home helper workers union tried to establish itself just before the introduction of the LTCI System. As of 2002 the All-Japan Prefectural and Municipal Workers Union (*Zen nihon jichidantai rengokai*) had 23,000 home helpers, but compared to other job areas this unionization rate has been low.

Political condition in the 1990s

The political background to the Gold Plan

There were political circumstances behind the creation of the Gold Plan. From the mid-1980s the Liberal Democratic Party government introduced a value-added tax in order to try and stabilize finances. However, the Japanese people reacted strongly to this rise in taxes and, with the failure to introduce the value-added tax (sales tax) as the trigger, Yasuhiro Nakasone's government (1982–87) resigned in 1987. Following on from this, the Noboru Takeshita government (1987–89) managed to successfully introduce value-added tax (consumption tax) at 3% in April 1989 after a hard-line vote in the Diet.

At the same time, the government was required to explain why it was necessary to introduce a consumption tax. It repeated that there was a need to make preparations for the coming aging of society and to ensure adequate financial resources. While advocating the idea of 'the Japanese-style social welfare model' and arguing that the burden for care should be borne by families, after the introduction of the consumption tax the Liberal Democratic Party had no choice but to submit its proposals for the Gold Plan.

In addition, the dramatic increase in medical expenditure had arisen as an issue, and long stays in hospital after treatment was completed (social admissions) was identified as one cause for the steep hike in costs.

The principle behind the Gold Plan was to enhance in-home welfare services. A home care support center was established in every junior high school district (with populations of approximately 16,000) and these were expected to function as in-home care access consultation points. The idea of constructing an in-home care system in each small district came largely from the Scandinavian countries.

From the beginning to the middle of the 1990s, there was a boom in sending municipal workers, care workers, and ordinary citizens to Sweden and Denmark to observe how the welfare systems worked there. From the learning gained about the system in Scandinavian countries, some municipalities set the goal of establishing independent home helpers who were able to respond twenty-four hours a day. At the time, in Scandinavian countries twenty-four-hour home help services were widespread and available to everybody. Nevertheless, in Japan, where there were no home help services on weekends or at night, achieving this seemed like a distant dream.

A non-Liberal Democratic Party coalition government and the LTCI idea

There was a complete transformation in the 1990s in the situation surrounding care policy, which until then had been devalued even by the government. In Japan, where the outsourcing of care had hardly moved forward at all, many researchers have made an analysis of the political situation of the time to try and understand what led to a social solution to the problem of care being pursued.

The mid-1990s was a unique period in Japan's political history. As a result of the 1993 lower house (House of Representatives) general election, which led to the birth of an eight-party non-Liberal Democratic Party coalition,[12] the Liberal Democratic Party became the opposition party for the first time since it was established in 1955. It returned to government in June 1994, in coalition with the Social Democratic Party and the New Party SAKIGAKE. It was obliged to work with these two parties that were not only interested in social security issues, but less wedded to familism. The period from 1993 to 1998 was exceptional in terms of Japanese politics and it was one where proposing and implementing a new care policy was relatively easy. For example, it was in 1994 that the idea of the LTCI System was first proposed by the Ministry of Health and Welfare. It was within the Ministry that a study group[13] was established to look into elderly care and the idea of supporting independence was first launched; further, in order to amass necessary financial resources, there was advocacy for the introduction of a new care insurance system.

For trade unions and their members, elderly care had also emerged as a serious issue and was much discussed. The Japanese Trade Union Confederation (Rengo)[14] reported the results of its own investigations in 1995, and this received public attention. The research targeted family carers of elderly parents. The research revealed the difficult conditions facing those involved in family-based care, both as providers and recipients. The research showed that 34.6% of family carers who responded to the survey felt that their elderly parents were hateful, and 49.6% of family carers had some experiences of abuse (Rengo 1995). While it was widely believed at the time that family care was the ideal model, the research made it clear that it was not necessarily the case.

For feminism, the care issue was a problem shared by all women and it led to the cooperation of full-time housewives and working women whose interests had appeared to stand in opposition. The previously mentioned Women's Association for the Better Aging Society is a civil society group that advocates for the improvement of policy concerning elderly care, and it brought together to the same debating table feminists calling for women's independence and ordinary housewives who were giving thought to the problem of elderly care. The argument that most users of care services, the care workers themselves, and those suffering under the burden of care in the home were women was highly persuasive and led to cooperation between women, whereas cooperation previously had been on the basis of whether they participated directly in the paid labor market or not.

In addition, there was increased reciprocal activity between the Ministry of Health and Welfare, the municipalities, and civil society. Municipalities proactively held symposiums and study meetings on the care issue, and listened to the voices of civil society activists and groups.

While the Liberal Democratic Party was in coalition with the Social Democratic Party, there had been a loosening of the hitherto line of familism in the government and its agencies. During this period, the Ministry of Health and Welfare had sought to establish a position of superiority and to gain ground in pushing forward the socialization of elderly care to some degree. At the same time feminist activism set as one of its goals the liberation of women from the burden of elderly care. While it was not clear whether all involved had exactly the same goals, they were all aiming in roughly the same direction.

Discussion of cash benefits

The LTCI bill was initially scrapped in 1996, but was later revived and successfully passed through the Diet, Japan's bicameral national legislature, in 1998. Following on from this, just as preparations were advancing throughout the country in readiness for implementation of the LTCI System in April 2000, there was a resurgence of familism. In October 1999—five months before the system was to be implemented—the Liberal Democratic Party Policy Research Council stated that Japan should not create a system that would destroy the 'fine custom of children caring for their parents.' In addition, it suggested the introduction of cash benefits for families caring for elderly parents. However, Japanese feminists, the Ministry of Health and Welfare, and local municipalities did not accept the introduction of cash payments. Feminists were angry at this attempt to halt the socialization of elderly care.

The Ministry of Health and Welfare and local municipalities were also angry that, after pushing ahead and setting up service infrastructure as far as they had, they were suddenly having the ladder taken away from underneath them. As with the case of Germany, there was concern that the introduction of cash benefits would result in the majority of beneficiaries taking this option and there would be insufficient finances to maintain the LTCI System.

In the Scandinavian countries there is a system where family members involved in caring can receive cash benefits. In Norway such a system has existed in some municipalities since 1960. Within the Norwegian Social Services Law, municipalities provide respite and a care allowance for families that carry out heavy-level care work. The care allowance is taxable. Furthermore, in 1988 the care allowance became institutionalized in the Municipal Medical Insurance Law and Norway expanded informal care to a higher degree than in the other Nordic countries (Wærness 1987). In 2003 there were 1850 people throughout the country receiving care allowances.

Two-thirds of the beneficiaries of care allowances in Norway are women (Wærness 1987), but in Japan, where familism is strong and equal opportunities between men and women have been slow to be realized, and where the volume of care services is extremely low, there was considerable anxiety that the introduction of a care allowance would ossify women as the bearers of the burden of care. Many people did not think that cash benefits would become a new alternative to improve freedom of choice in Japan.

Home help and new public management (2000–)

The character of the LTCI System

Various care providers and freedom of choice

The LTCI System was introduced in April 2000. With the introduction of the LTCI System, there was a dramatic increase in users of home help services. Table 3.3 offers a comparison of the number of care service users before and after the introduction of LTCI. This shows that over a period of eight years, the number of users of in-home services[15] increased more than two times. It means that the number of home help users also increased. Historically, such a dramatic increase in the use of in-home care services had not occurred before. The background to this increase is the expansion of middle-income users who had previously found it particularly difficult to access care services.

Article 2 of the LTCI Law (*Kaigo hoken hō*) states that 'care insurance services must be provided by a variety of organizations' and it promotes a diversification of providers. Before the introduction of the LTCI System, home help services were provided by social welfare corporations[16] and councils of social welfare,[17] which were commissioned by local municipalities. In addition, there were some home help services provided by private for-profit companies, but they charged high prices and did not contribute to an increase in users. What happened, then, after the introduction of the LTCI System? Table 3.4 shows the diversification in in-home service providers.

Table 3.3: Increase in users of care services (2001 and 2009)

Number of users	2001	2009	Rate of increase
Facility-based services	613,000	839,000	37%
In-home services	1,337,000	2,839,000	112%
(Home help service	518,000	1,154,000	123%)

Note: statistics come from April 2001 and April 2009. Users of home help service are included in the users of in-home services.

Source: Based on Ministry of Health, Labour, and Welfare (Japan) 2001, 2009.

Table 3.4: Trends in the number of home help service providers (2001 and 2007)

By corporate status	2001	2007	Rate of increase
Social welfare corporation (incl. Council of social welfare)	4,894	5,592	14.3%
Non-profit medical corporation	1,245	1,522	22.2%
Public interest corporations	236	257	8.9%
For-profit corporation	3,959	11,392	187.7%
Non-profit organizations	362	1,242	243.1%
Agricultural cooperative societies	952	1,189	27.7%
Cooperative societies	584	746	40.0%
Local governments	228	157	–31.1%
Others	136	161	18.4%
Total	11,644	21,069	80.9%

Note: statistics come from October 2001 and October 2007.

Source: Based on Ministry of Health, Labour, and Welfare (Japan) 2001, 2007.

This includes day care and short stay services; however, it is noteworthy that for-profit companies and NPOs expanded home help services.

It is a positive result of the new system that the amount of service has dramatically increased. But rapid change has brought some serious problems and challenges.

A massive scandal arose with the rapid increase in private for-profit organizations providing care. The company COMSN[18] held a 2% share of the care market nationwide and expanded its operations with the introduction of the LTCI System. Disregarding the commercial viability of what it was doing, the company advanced service provision in less-densely populated areas. However, in the summer of 2007 it was discovered to have been making bogus claims for remuneration for care provision. At the same time, it was found that it had engaged in other wrong-doing, such as not observing the standards set for the deployment of staff. Ultimately, the company was forced to discontinue business (Chapter 6).

The Scandinavian model of home help system that started in the 1990s has almost disappeared in Japan. Highly motivated municipalities introduced the Scandinavian model of home help and tried to support the frail elderly at home twenty-four hours a day, 365 days a year. The Scandinavian model of home help does not work well in a freedom-of-choice system like the LTCI. It is quite difficult for municipalities and providers to organize a twenty-four-hour home help network in a small area because each elderly person can choose his or her own favorite provider, even from another area.

Needs assessment in a purchaser–provider model

In the period that Christensen (2005: 41–2) refers to as 'late modern outputs,' Norway added new administrative procedures between care providers and care users. Called the *purchaser–provider model*, it resulted in the formalizing and standardizing of care services.

The Japanese LTCI System also introduced the purchaser–provider model. As a result of the LTCI System, the framework of needs assessment and care management was brought to Japan for the first time. Each municipality has a responsibility of needs assessment in theory, but the Ministry of Health, Labour, and Welfare controls almost everything. In contrast to Norway and Sweden, where variations exist between municipalities, in Japan there is a unified system for the whole country and there is a strong hue of centralization.

The needs assessment that occurs within the Japanese LTCI System is referred to as 'certification of long-term care need' (*yō kaigo nintei*) and is carried out on the basis of a questionnaire checklist (of seventy-four items)[19] that is unified across the country. The first stage of the needs assessment (which has seven needs levels and an independent level) is done by computer and involves a calculation of the time needed for care (see Table 3.5). On the basis of this first-stage needs assessment, there is a second stage where a Committee for the Certification of Need (*nintei sinsakai*), made up of doctors and other health professionals, finally determines the necessary care level.

A new category of certification was introduced in April 2006. Approximately 40% to 50% of elderly who had been assessed at 'Care level 1' were reassessed as 'Requiring support 1' or 'Requiring support 2.' It means that the number of elderly who are assessed at 'Care level 1' has decreased.

In addition, the Ministry of Health, Labour, and Welfare changed the format of the assessment questionnaire in April 2009. As a result of

Table 3.5: Assessment category and benefit in the LTCI System (from April 2006)

Level of assessment	Monthly benefit	User's fee
Independent	0 yen	0 yen
Requiring support 1	49,700 yen	4,970 yen
Requiring support 2	104,000 yen	10,400 yen
Care level 1	165,800 yen	16,580 yen
Care level 2	194,800 yen	19,480 yen
Care level 3	267,500 yen	26,750 yen
Care level 4	306,000 yen	30,600 yen
Care level 5	358,300 yen	35,830 yen

Source: Based on Ministry of Health, Labour, and Welfare (Japan) 2009.

assessment reform in 2006 and again in 2009, elderly who needed a modest level of support such as cleaning, washing, or cooking, had their services reduced. These assessment reforms have been criticized by researchers and journalists because they have reduced care services.

The government is understandably concerned about the prospect of further dramatic increases in the LTCI budget.[20] While it was 3.6 trillion yen in 2000, it increased to 7.2 trillion yen by 2008. The Ministry of Health, Labour, and Welfare has tried to reduce long-term care benefits through assessment reforms.

Care managers as new specialists in the LTCI System

Once the certification of long-term care need is completed, care management takes place. The position of a care manager who creates a care plan is a new one created through the establishment of the LTCI System. There are two notable characteristics about the care manager in the Japanese context when compared to other countries.

First, there is the care manager license. The qualification of care manager is awarded as a result of a national examination; however, even non-care specialists such as pharmacists and acupuncturists can gain the license. In other words, in Japan it is not necessary to be a specialist in elderly care to become a care manager. In 2003, 300,000 care manager licenses were awarded.

Second, generally in Japan the care manager is employed by a care service provider. As a result, there is a risk that the care manager will create a care plan that prioritizes services provided by the organization to which he or she belongs rather than manage services necessary for the user. A number of studies have pointed to the difficulty of establishing the independence of the care manager under the current system.

Care managers have an important position in relation to the elderly and their families. Care users are supposed to talk to their care managers about their needs, and not to the home helpers. Home helpers cannot work for users outside the care plan that a care manager has made. Under the LTCI Law (Article 8-2), the work of home helpers is to help with bathing, toileting, eating, and other tasks for daily life. Advice and consultation are no longer the responsibility of home helpers, but are part of care managers' work. Home helpers are supposed to concentrate on the more practical work.

Service reduction in the 2005 LTCI reform

The reduction of housework support

Christensen notes that with the purchaser–provider model there is authorization of the types and level of care services to be provided to the homes of the elderly, but this is done by somebody who in reality does not actually provide these care services. In other words, there is a clear separation of responsibilities between the person who decides the volume and type of service and the home helper. As a result, there is an increase in the tasks over which the home helper has no determination.

The Japanese LTCI System recognizes two types of home help. First, 'physical care' (*shintai kaigo*), which involves operative care to help the user in daily life, in particular with washing, dressing, toileting, and diaper changing. This costs around 2310 yen (US$25.37/EUR16.91) per half-hour, of which the user pays 10% and the LTCI covers 90%.

The second type of home help recognized by the government is 'daily life support' (*seikatsu shien*).[21] Here the home helper carries out some of the household chores necessary for daily life that the user is unable to do for her or himself, such as cleaning, laundry, food preparation, and shopping. This service costs around 2080 yen per half-hour, of which the user bears 10% of the cost and the LTCI bears 90%.

The scope of housework support has arisen as a point of debate. The scope of housework support has been stipulated by the Ministry of Health, Labour, and Welfare and the kind of activities that are not recognized can loosely be summed up as follows.

First, any activities that do not directly support the user fall outside the Ministry's designation of daily life support. In particular, it is judged that it is appropriate for the home helpers to carry out any activities that serve to make life more convenient for the family. As an example of such activities, the Ministry cites carrying out laundry, food preparation, or shopping that is for anyone other than the user, the cleaning of any room other than the one occupied by the user, or serving guests who come to the house.

Second, activities that do not support the lifestyle of the user also fall outside the Ministry's definition of home help. Examples offered by the Ministry include weeding the garden, watering the flowers, pet care, and window cleaning. The Ministry also states that the user must not request additional activities connected to the main task such as 'tidying up the whole kitchen after doing the cooking' or 'throwing out the rubbish after doing the shopping.'

As other examples, when it comes to the care activity of accompanying an elderly person on a hospital trip, the home helper cannot be asked to carry out care activities within the hospital; and, in the house of an elderly couple, food preparation should only be for the elderly user and not the spouse. Since the revision of the LTCI Law in 2005, guidance[22] from the Ministry of Health, Labour, and Welfare on home helper activities has become stricter.

Home-visit services to prevent the need for care

As a result of the revision of the LTCI System in 2005, the importance of prevention and rehabilitation as a central part of policy has been made clear. Along with this, a new category of home help services has been added to the benefits menu, that of 'home-visit services to prevent the need for care' (*Kaigo yobō houmon kaigo*).

This new category of services can be provided to those elderly who, on the basis of Certification of Long-term Care Need, are designated as 'Requiring support 1' or 'Requiring support 2' (see Table 3.5). They are entitled to home help services once or twice a week and the care fee that they have to pay to the provider is relatively cheap compared to that of in-home care services. Under the law, 'in-home care services' offer 'care' (*sewa*) in daily life, whereas 'home-visit services to prevent the need for care' provides 'support' (*shien*) with daily life. With 'home-visit services to prevent the need for care,' the emphasis is on allowing the care users to do as much for themselves as they can while keeping an eye on this process.

As a result of the introduction of the 'home-visit services to prevent the need for care,' there has been a decrease in the use of the hitherto home help service. In September 2005, immediately after the system was revised, there were 1,090,112 users of home help services, but in September 2006 there were 822,556 users and in October 2007 there were 738,793 users (Ministery of Health, Labour and Welfare, 2005, 2006, and 2007). This means that in the first year after the revision the number of in-home care users declined by 304,800. This is the first time there had been a decrease in the use of home help services since the system of 'home servants for the elderly' was established more than fifty years ago.

On the one hand, during this same period the number of users of 'home-visit services to prevent the need for care' increased from 159,791 in 2006 to 306,458 in 2007. From the perspective of the volume of service provided and the cost, there was a cut in the level of home help services.

A final overview of the transition in home help

The aim of this chapter was to draw on Christensen's concept of the modernization of home help and Wærness's concept of the rationality of care to make a comparison between the development processes in Japan and Norway in order to clarify differences and similarities.

Table 3.6 shows an overview of the transition of home help in Japan. There is some similarity in both countries. At the beginning of home help services, it was said that a charitable mind and passion were necessary to work as a home helper. But this work has concentrated on more practical work than talking with care users.

Below, I summarize the key points developed in this chapter focusing particularly on the following: the character of home help development in Japan, the short period of *modernization* of home help in Japan, and challenges of home help in Norway and Japan.

The special characteristics of the development of home help in Japan

A number of special characteristics can be highlighted concerning the development of home help in Japan in the period 1960 to 1980. In Japan the institutionalization of home help services occurred very early, at the beginning of the 1960s, but through to the 1990s use of home helpers in ordinary homes was almost non-existent. The expansion of home help in Norway occurred in the 1970s and the particular characteristics that we can point to here are the systematization and bureaucratization of services. In Japan, however, where home help was introduced in the form of 'home servants for the elderly,' services were strongly associated with poor relief policy and there was little expansion in volume of usage.

Four reasons have been offered for why home help services did not expand during this initial period. During the 1970s the rate of aging in Japanese society was still low, at around 8%, and more than 70% of elderly were co-residing with their adult children. It is thought that the pre-war teaching that welfare services are for those elderly who are all alone in the

Table 3.6: Transition of home help in Japan

Name	Contents of work	Care users
Home help service outline (Rōjin katei hōshiin jigyō unei yōkō)*: 1962*		
Home servants for the elderly (*rōjin katei hōshiin*)	Two kinds of services are included. 1. Housekeeping (*kaji*) and care (*kaigo*). Care for eating, laundry, cleaning, and other kinds of care. 2. Consultation (*sōdan*) and advice (*jyogen*) for daily life. 'Charity mindset is necessary for home helpers' (White Paper, 1962).	Households with elderly who are physically or mentally handicapped and need social assistance (free service).
Revision of home help service outline (Kaitei Rōjin katei hōshiin jigyō unei yōkō)*: 1970*		
Home servants for the elderly (*rōjin katei hōshiin*)	As in 1962. 'Home helper has a role to talk with elderly, as a so called consultant of daily life' (White Paper, 1969).	Low-income bedridden elderly who need daily life support and have no family to take care of (free service).
Revision of home help service outline (Kaitei Rōjin katei hōshi in jigyō unei yōkō)*: 1982*		
Home servants for the elderly (*rōjin katei hōshiin*)	As in 1962. 'Home helpers are required to be physically and mentally healthy, having passion and understanding of elderly care, and having ability and experience of housekeeping, elderly care, and advising' (Article 8, The outline, 1982).	Bedridden elderly who are over sixty-five years (fee depends on income of household).
Revision of home help service outline (Kaitei Rōjin katei hōshi in jigyō unei yōkō) *and Gold Plan: 1989*		
Home helper (*hōmu herupa-*)	Three types of home help services 1. Physical care (*shintai kaigo*). Aid with washing, dressing, toileting, diaper changing. 2. Housework support (*kaji enjo*). Cleaning, laundry, food preparation, shopping. 3. Consultation (*sōdan*) and advice (*jyogen*) for daily life. Home helpers' grade system was introduced in 1994. Level 1 course is for home helpers who will work as managers (230 hours). Level 2 course is for home helpers who will work in all kinds of home help services (130-hour course). Level 3 course is for home helpers who will work only doing housekeeping (50-hour course).	Bedridden elderly who are over sixty-five years (fee depends on income of household).

Table 3.6: continued

Name	Contents of work	Care users
LTCI Law: 2000		
Visiting care worker (*hōmon kaigoin*)	Three types of home help services: 1. Physical care (*shintai kaigo*). Aid with washing, dressing, toileting, diaper changing. 2. Housework support (*kaji enjo*). Cleaning, laundry, food preparation, shopping. 3. Mixed model (a mix of 1 and 2 above)	Insured elderly who need full-time care due to confinement to bed or dementia, or those who do not need full-time care but need daily life assistance (10% co-payment).
LTCI Law (revision of remuneration for care service in 2003): 2003		
Visiting care worker (*hōmon kaigoin*)	Two types of home help services. 'Housework support' (*kaji enjoy*) has changed its name to 'daily life support' (*seikatsu sien*). Mixed model was abolished.	As in 2000.
LTCI Law (revision of the Law of the LTCI in 2005): 2006		
Visiting care worker (*hōmon kaigoin*)	'Home-visit services to prevent the need for care' (*kaigo yobō hōmon kaigo*) for the elderly who are assessed as 'Requiring support 1' and 'Requiring support 2.'	As in 2000.

world and without economic means served to slow down the development of home help in Japan. Second, in the private sector, enterprises dispatching housekeepers stood in competition with home help services. As the wages of housekeepers were relatively low and their services could also be used by other members of the elderly person's household, this reduced the incentive to develop public home help services. Third, there was also strong resistance to outsourcing care work. It was thought that the dispatch of 'home servants for the elderly' would result in a weakening of relations within the family. Finally, there was the stance of the Japanese government towards social security. The government policy of a 'Japanese-style welfare' model that appeared in the 1970s with the oil crisis encouraged families to take up the burden of elderly care.

Modernization of home help

In Japan's case, Christensen's *modernization* period can be said to be the 1990s, when the Gold Plan was instituted. This period is shorter compared with Norway, and it is difficult to identify exactly the cut-off point. But during this period we can find some of the same characteristics as Norway's period in that every municipality throughout Japan had to draw up a plan to institute care services and home help started to be organized. At the same time, care work started to be professionalized. Care workers were encouraged to have professional training and social worker, care worker, and home help qualification levels one to three were instituted in the care field. However, there was an increase in home helpers who were employed on the basis of the register model without stable employment conditions and the professionalization process did not result in an elevation of their social status.

Comparing this situation with that of Norway, the period of modernization in Japan was short. As a result, the organization and professionalization of home help ended up being cut short and we can speculate that this prevented home help receiving the social status of being an occupation in Japan.

Christensen's *late modern period* began in the late 1990s in Japan and is symbolized by the LTCI System. The establishment of the LTCI System signifies the safeguarding of elderly care and was welcomed as significant in terms of the public funding of care services. In reality there was a dramatic increase in the use of home help services. However, the same system strengthened the strict management of care work in terms of working time, content, and costs.

With the dramatic increase in service usage over the previous five years, the revisions in 2005 reflected the heightened alarm over future financing of the LTCI. Greater emphasis was placed on the necessity of prevention and rehabilitation to ensure that care would not be required, even by those who are elderly. The menu of insurance benefits increased to include rehabilitation and training, which at the same time made it more difficult for elderly users co-residing with family to receive home help. In 2006 the volume of home help declined on previous years. Since the institutionalization of home help in Japan in 1962, service use had increased continuously, even though there are differences depending on the period, so this was a new phenomenon. At the same time, it became more difficult to secure home resources in the care field and the government began to look into the possibility of drawing on labor from other parts of Asia.

Challenges facing home-help services

As a result of the implementation of the Gold Plan in the 1990s and the LTCI System in 2000, home help was organized and professionalized in Japan. This modernization process was critical in the expansion and normalization of home help in Japan. Debate about the sustainability of the system began, the concepts of rehabilitation and prevention were debated, and there have been demands for the rationalization of home help. There have been cut backs in the content of home help and time usage and a strengthening of the management of the system. With demands for impersonal work and high turnover rates, there is now a shortage of home helpers. The bureaucratic dilemma that Wærness indicated can now be seen within the development process of home help in Japan.

When care work is carried out by people with formal employment relations, interaction at the care site is subject to the management of a third party. The subjects of management are not only the care worker's movements and emotions, but stretch to the emotions of the person receiving the care. The characteristics of modern organization that accelerates control by non-human techniques such as efficiency, computability, and predictability are even permeating the nature of personal human services.

If we return to Wærness's concept of the rationality of care, the same methods cannot be used as with the production of manufactured goods when attempting to rationalize work that is tied in with human emotion. What has to be done to achieve a balance between providing a sustainable care system and high standard home help? On this point, there is shared ground between the challenges faced in Norway and those in Japan.

Chapter 4
Long-Term Care Insurance, Marketization, and Quality of Care: 'Good Time Living'

Reiko Abe Auestad

Introduction[1]

Given the changes both in demographic structure and in women's expectations, in Japanese society in the 1990s the government realized that it could no longer rely on the *Japanese-style welfare society* to manage the overwhelming task of an ageing society.[2] Meeting the demands of the rapidly ageing population obviously meant a use of greater resources than just *families*. Launching a program for reforming the basic structure of social welfare (*shakai fukushi kiso kōzō kaikaku*), in 2000 the government introduced the Long-Term Care Insurance (LTCI) System (*Kaigo hoken seido*), a social insurance system aimed at the rapid development of various types of care provision with the help of market forces. Considered by many as a step in the direction towards a *socialization of care*, high expectations mounted. In the summary of the overall program, the concept behind the reform was stipulated as follows: it is based on the idea that 'social welfare should help an individual live an independent life suited to his/her own needs with dignity' and aims at an 'individual's independence, choice and a social service of high quality' (Katō 2002: 11).

The LTCI is 45% financed by insurance fees,[3] 45% financed by the state and the municipalities, and 10% by the users themselves. The users receive needs certification for the amount of care approved based on an assessment by the Committee for the Certification of Need, a committee made up of doctors and other health professionals. Based on this, the user can decide with the help of a care manager which services to purchase, and from whom. The providers of services and care management can be either non-profit organizations or for-profit agencies, and the type of services offered can vary from housework assistance, physical assistance, visiting nurse, and bathing service to the use of day center and short stay services.

The new insurance system thus lets the market establish a network of welfare-related institutions of various origin, status, and size that participate in providing care. The idea is to create social services of high quality by promoting competition. Critics of the reform have, however, argued from the outset that this strategy of marketization (quasi-marketization) would result in differentiation among the clients in terms of quality and amount of care that they receive.[4] Since the prices of the services are fixed independently of the users' incomes, even the 10% fees would be too costly for those with low incomes, while the wealthiest can buy more services than the LTCI entitles them to by paying 100% of the expenses.[5] Paradoxically, it is the wealthiest who can afford to pay who receive the most public subsidies. It has also been pointed out that there will be regional differences because private providers will not establish their businesses in places where they are not sustainable or profitable.

Eight years since the start of the LTCI, many Japanese scholars and observers, especially those who favor the state-sponsored, standardized Nordic model of welfare, have remained skeptical about the principle of marketization (quasi-marketization). In one volume of the six-volume collection on care that came out in 2008, Naohiko Jinno argues that the LTCI only caters to the demands of the wealthy middle class, while Noriko Kurube rather categorically labels the LTCI as inspired by 'the Anglo Saxon model of new public management' (Jinno 2008: 19–20; Kurube 2008: 49).

In the meantime, there are some pragmatists who recognize positive effects of marketization on the quality of care (Hiraoka 2008: 132). Kōichi Hiraoka in the same volume notes that it is generally agreed that the LTCI has had a positive effect on the quality of care, particularly in terms of flexibility in responding to the demands of clients. In the discussions in the 1990s prior to implementation of the LTCI, there was a fear that the LTCI would result in the spread of poor-quality services, but, he points out, this has turned out not to be the case at all. Hiraoka also argues that the current problems related to the quality of care in the LTCI are not necessarily directly related to marketization per se. It has, rather, more to do with other factors such as the laxness of the regulations concerning the care staff, the low salaries of care workers, inadequate training and education, inappropriate systems of care management, and an ambiguity with regard to responsibility in regulating providers' activities (Hiraoka 2008: 133).

Outside Japan, in 2002 John Creighton Campbell gave by far the most optimistic and positive assessment of the LTCI System albeit with a qualification that 'the experiment was still in early days' (Campbell 2002: 9). Drawing attention to the size of the program 'estimated even officially as running over USD [United State dollars] 50 billion a year when fully implemented' (Campbell 2002: 9), he foresaw the possibility that Japan would make 'a quantum leap ahead of' other industrialized nations in terms of the 'care for the frail elderly.' He continued, saying that this is not only a massive transfer of financial responsibility from family to government or 'socialization of care.' The way care is delivered is, on the one hand, radically separated from the family by covering only formal services rather than family care allowances, as in Germany, and, on the other, is much more individual choice-oriented than the controlled and bureaucratic (some might say paternalistic) approach in the Nordic countries (Campbell 2002: 10). Campbell seemed to suggest here that the LTCI might be thought of as an alternative social welfare model that would move in a third or even fourth space between state-socialized care (Nordic) and a market forces neo-liberalist model (Anglo-American), which would distinguish itself at the same time from the German corporate model that Esping-Andersen once categorized Japan as belonging to (Esping-Andersen 1990). As I will touch upon in more detail later, the point Campbell made about 'socialization of care' is one shared by many Japanese feminists in their assessment of the LTCI.

To sum up, many of the pro and con arguments revolve around the effect of marketization (quasi-marketization) on the quality of care, and on the universal availability of care—extremely important issues in the international debate on the various social welfare models. As Noriko Kurube and many others have illustrated, the debate on marketization has taken place in the Nordic countries as well. In the neo-liberalistic political climate in the 1990s, many municipalities in the Nordic countries started giving consignments to private providers. The difference with the Japanese system, however, is that its use of private providers is motivated by the need to increase effectiveness in the public sector and does not necessarily aim at giving clients a greater possibility to choose. Even in municipalities that give clients freedom of choice, the freedom is often quite nominal in the case of senior housing because the demand often overwhelmingly exceeds the supply (Yayoi Saito, pers. comm., August 15, 2008).

With the varied assessments of the LTCI as a backdrop, I would like to examine a concrete example of the possible effect of marketization on the quality of care in Tsuru no sato, a recently established so-called 'licensed private senior housing' (*yūryō rōjin hōmu*) on the outskirts of Tokyo. My interest in private senior housing is due to its great potential in playing a role in realizing the socialization of care, albeit only for the middle class to begin with. Partly because the number of government-operated long-term care facilities (such as '*tokuyō* special nursing homes') is very limited, the demand for licensed private senior housing is increasing.[6] Even though it is called *private senior housing*, it does not necessarily fit the extravagant image the term used to give, or may still give in other places (such as in the United States).[7] Their residents have to pay facility fees and bear other necessary living expenses on their own, but the care expenses are subsidized by the LTCI. In other words, the cost of living in such facilities has become much more affordable. Private senior housing of various types, which before the introduction of the LTCI was out of reach for the middle class or simply did not exist, has become a real alternative.[8]

Since home help within the LTCI, even for the most heavily dependent, is often not sufficient and presupposes considerable help from the family, affordable private senior homes can play a significant role in relieving the family/women of the burden of care. In the Japanese cultural context, where the women traditionally have been made to feel guilty unless they yield their utmost as primary caregivers, and where living space often is limited, reasonably priced private senior facilities may hold the key to a real socialization of care.[9] I have chosen Tsuru no sato because it is representative in the sense that it caters to middle-class clients and demonstrates a rather successful case of marketization by creating its own, distinct profile. Before analyzing the quality of care in Tsuru no sato, however, I would like to summarize the relevant aspects of the Western feminist debate on the dependency critique in order to give my analysis a comparative and feminist perspective.

An ethic of care that embraces dependency

With an awareness that equality has eluded women because they have traditionally occupied *inequitable positions* at home and have been excluded from the general reference class for humanity, many feminists in the West have been engaged in the so-called *critiques of equality* from various perspectives.[10] Inspired by these strands of feminist thinking, while also refining her position, Eva Kittay elaborates on what she calls *dependency critique* in an attempt to formulate a new ethic of care that takes into account the complex challenges involved in dealing with the necessarily asymmetrical, inequitable positions of the dependents and the caregivers. Arguing that undisputed, universal concepts such as equality and rationality must be rethought and relativized in a care situation in light of the necessarily specific relationship between each dependent and caregiver, she emphasizes that the 'moral obligations between the parties are not the general obligations,' but special ones 'particular to the individual in that relationship;' an ethic of care therefore 'understands moral reasoning to be contextual and responsive rather than a calculus performed on rights or utilities', and 'centers not on impartial judgments, but on judgments partial to participants within a caring relation' (Kittay 1999: 53–4).

In the Nordic context, this line of argument resonates well with that of a Norwegian feminist researcher, Kari Wærness, who has been advocating a redefinition of *rationality* in the care situation—something that she coins a *rationality of caring*—since the beginning of the 1980s. In contradistinction to the kind of abstract scientific rationality that had long been overemphasized in the Western discourse on public management, Wærness elaborates on the importance of the down-to-earth, pragmatic rationality anchored in 'what most of us in our everyday life perceive as the essential values in a caring relationship' (Wærness 1984: 187). The rationality of caring sometimes commands us to pass emotive and *impartial* evaluations of the overall situation, and to take actions that may even go counter to what is most commonly thought of as *rational*. Using empirical examples from the motherly care of the child, which operates 'on the level of the particular and individual,' she argues that there is something fundamental in the nature of care work that resists generalization and standardization, and, in that sense, the rationality of caring is not only different but also 'to some degree contradictory to the scientific rationality' (Wærness 1984: 197, 195).

Wærness's rationality of caring is a critique of the type of rationality that she believes 'dominates in the planning of, and research on the public service apparatus' in the Nordic countries, and the bureaucratic, fragmented, and impersonal ways in which services in the public sector are being provided (Wærness 1999: 54–5).

In concrete terms, the main address of her criticism in Norway has been the home help services because that is where the problems have been most visible. Bureaucratic standardization in the name of rationality has led to an increasing division of labor. At the same time a lack of communication between the decision-making and task-implementing apparatus, and among the task-implementing care workers themselves, has resulted in a fragmentation of the care work itself (Wærness 2008: 369–70). A district nurse in Oslo told me that an average user of the home help service would, in the course of a week, receive assistance from up to fifteen different care workers in various capacities and with various areas of specialization, which makes it difficult for any one person to have an overview of the client's condition and to cultivate the contextual and responsive care relationship with the client (Larsen 2008). Another nurse in Oslo touched upon a similar problem of rigidity in the division of labor in a private care home, St Halvardshjemmet, where he works (Goonetilleke 2008). Even when nurses are understaffed due to illness, some assistant care workers adamantly refuse to give patients medicine because it is the nurse's job, not theirs.

Japanese feminists have been mostly concerned with cultural factors and circumstances surrounding the care situation that have prevented *socialization of care* rather than with the quality of care itself,[11] and not many have actively participated in the Western debate on the relational/contextual nature of care.[12] I nevertheless find the relational/contextual nature of care as it has been discussed by Western feminists relevant in my analysis because it finds certain resonance with the principle of care upheld in Tsuru no sato, as I will return to later, and most likely in many other care institutions in Japan.

It should be pointed out, however, that Kari Wærness's rationality of care demands that it should not be exercised at the expense of the *self-sufficiency* of the client, a point that currently does not seem to be emphasized to the same extent in the Japanese discourse on care (even though it is mentioned in the 2006 LTCI reform, it is more motivated by a need to reduce the level of spending than by concern for the quality of care). Wærness writes:

> There should be at the same time an implicit demand that services and help should be given in such a way as not to weaken the care receiver's ability to take care for himself/herself. If possible, it should even strengthen it. It is humiliating for the care receiver if the caregiver either underestimates or overestimates his/her independence. It therefore requires on the part of the caregiver both a closeness and the ability to understand the care-receiver's situation so as to give care without denigrating the care-receiver's dignity (my translation, Wærness 1999: 49).

In Wærness's scheme, self-sufficiency is a premise that ought to be maintained in a care-giving relationship at all times. A new relational ethic of care based on pragmatic rationality should not override the golden principle of self-sufficiency. The obvious challenge in the marketized care of the elderly, such as in Japan, is that wealthy *clients* can define their own vulnerability, if they are so disposed, and may neglect the principle of self-sufficiency. Theoretically speaking, wealthy clients can use their financial power to buy self-sufficiency rather than dependency, but, as I will discuss later, there seems to be a culturally influenced factor that makes many of the middle-class residents of care homes more disposed to dependency rather than self-sufficiency.

Kittay indirectly touches upon the same *money* problem in discussing vulnerability. Critically referring to Robert Goodin's model of vulnerability, Kittay problematizes the definition and assessment of the recipient's vulnerability and self-sufficiency. According to Goodin, '[w]hether or not the existing allocation of responsibilities itself has any moral warrant, it has made some people vulnerable to others; and that fact, if no other, provides a moral warrant for discharging those responsibilities' (Kittay 1999: 59; Goodin 1985: 125). Goodin thereby acknowledges the *pragmatic 'ought'* attached to the vulnerability claims, endorsing it as a necessary part of dependency care; one ought to help the vulnerable regardless of the circumstances.

Even as she acknowledges the 'moral pull of being in a relation with another who is vulnerable to one's actions' (Kittay 1999: 64), Kittay questions Goodin's insistence on treating 'the existing allocation of responsibilities' as a 'social fact.' She cites an example from Tony Morrison's novel, *Song of Solomon*, in which Circe, a black girl who is the only remaining servant of Miss Butler, the now destitute daughter of a formerly wealthy family, chooses to stay with Miss Butler despite the fact that Circe is free to leave. It all ends, however, with Miss Butler's suicide, which provokes indignation in Circe. Circe exclaims: 'I said she killed herself rather than do the work I'd been doing all my life!...Do you hear me? She saw the work I did all her days and died, you hear me, died rather than live like me' (Kittay 1999: 58).

Kittay uses Circe's statement to support her argument that 'false needs can be generated...within a relation of dependency,' and concludes, 'responding to the needs of another unjustly thrust upon us is, in itself, demeaning,' thereby discrediting the legitimacy of Goodin's model (Kittay 1999: 59). The upshot of Kittay's claim is that accepting 'the pragmatic ought leaves no place from which to challenge unfair allocations' of responsibilities of care work (Kittay 1999: 64). Even as I agree with Kittay in principle, I would point out that distinguishing *false needs* from *real needs* is no simple matter precisely because we are dealing with someone who is in a relation of dependency to us. And the question of marketization further complicates the assessment of the legitimacy of her/his moral claims.

Differences not only between paid and unpaid dependency work, but also among various types of paid dependency work in Japan, add to the complexity of assessing the 'inevitable variety of human interactions' (Kittay 1999: 15). In the Japanese context of the LTCI, therefore, many of the questions concerning the elusive quality of care that Kittay asks become especially pertinent. The *question of equality* fragments into *questions of equalities*: 'Equality *for whom*? Equality *by what measure*? Equality of *what*? Equal *to what*? Equal *to whom*?' (Kittay 1999: 5).

I will examine the various aspects of care as it is performed in Tsuru no sato with a focus on how the *rationality of care* (Wærness 1984) and the special characteristics of dependency work, such as responsiveness and connectedness (Kittay 1999), are encouraged or/and practiced, even as the coerced pragmatic ought sometimes may intervene negatively in the process, undermining self-sufficiency.

Tsuru no sato

Despite the fact that private senior housing facilities are owned by both for-profit agencies and NPOs, social welfare foundations, and cooperatives, the differences of expenses among them are moderate (except, of course, for those that specifically target upper-income seniors). As already noted, the care costs are equally subsidized by the LTCI (in other words, it is the cost of housing and living, which the LTCI does not cover, that differentiates their expenses). The prices of care services and the kind of care-related activities of the providers are also so tightly regulated that there is relatively little room for profit making. When one talks about the effect of marketization/market forces on the quality of care in these institutions, therefore, it does not necessarily involve profit-making motivations. It has more to do with the need to make their own profiles clearer to improve their images in the market.[13]

Tsuru no sato is operated by a social welfare foundation called Gasshōsen. Originally a temple, it is run by its own set of principles, some of which are clearly inspired by Buddhism. Developing what started out as a voluntary shelter for the homeless elderly into one of the first public homes right after the Second World War, the foundation has gradually expanded the range of services by building other facilities. It is only recently that it became engaged in building private senior housing such as Tsuru no sato, which opened in June 2004.[14] Tsuru no sato has created its own marketing profile by incorporating Mitsuru Haruyama's concept of *good time living* and his philosophy of management.

Mitsuru Haruyama and Tsuru no sato

Haruyama is a successful entrepreneur and an ardent spokesman for promoting paid dependency work to enhance the quality of living for the elderly and handicapped. He is, himself, deeply care dependent and has a heavy handicap. He was running a real estate agency when he was diagnosed with multiple sclerosis at the age of twenty-four. Trying to buy a wheelchair that accommodated his needs, he was shocked by the indifference and the lack of understanding on the part of those who were selling these products. This gave him an incentive to start his own business. Thirty years later he is paralyzed from the neck down, and is completely dependent on a wheelchair and other devices, as well as on help from others. Still, he is actively involved in the planning of projects dealing with dependency work in the broad sense. Featured among the 'Stars of Asia' in the June 3, 2003, issue of *Business Week*, he was 'the driving force behind Japan's first "mixed-living" community, which opened in a Tokyo suburb in May:' 'The $220 million complex, financed by Orix Corp., comprises 740 homes and apartments for families, assisted living facilities, and medical and day care for everyone from toddlers to the elderly' (Clifford 2003).

Interestingly, Haruyama writes in one of his internet sites that he learned his positive attitude towards old age late one night in Denmark in a pub crowded with old people. When he asked one man who was drinking into the early hours of the morning if he did not worry about his health, the old man replied that he would have plenty of time to rest when he dies, so he wouldn't worry. This episode inspired Haruyama to develop his own concept of life for the elderly, which he dubbed 'the concept of good time' (*guddo taimu no rinen*) and which can roughly be summarized as the enjoyment of life in old age. This Japanized English expression, *good time*, shows up frequently in the vocabulary of Haruyama's projects for the elderly. Old age in Japan has not been viewed as a stage of life to be enjoyed in a late night pub, but as a phase of life that should be endured with dignity in the care of one's family. It is a time with certain privileges in that one is allowed more indulgence, but it is also a quiet time before one's departure that should be lived with austerity and restraint.[15] And it is this view of old age that the Danish crowd at the pub subverted.

The building at Tsuru no sato has seven floors and consists of the assisted nursing home on the first, third, and fourth floors (the second floor is reserved for the heavily disabled) and a senior apartment complex on the fifth, sixth, and seventh floors. Each floor in the assisted nursing home consists of twenty-nine individual rooms, a common bathroom, a lounge, and a dining and living area with a reception, and staff quarters on each floor. Part of the first floor is reserved as a community floor, and has a spacious dining/restaurant area that can be converted into an entertainment hall if necessary, and several other common rooms and facilities (such as a beauty salon and a dental clinic). The administration office with care managers and nurses, as well as a clinic with two part-time, in-house doctors, is also located on the first floor. Residents in the senior apartments are generally more independent, but they can buy cleaning and care services, and are guaranteed the right to move into the nursing home by paying monthly fees. They can also eat at the restaurant or participate in the club activities, together with the residents of the nursing home, at an extra cost.[16]

In an interview for *Misora* (Winter 2006), a journal published by Haruyama's Orix Corporation, the manager of Tsuru no sato, Akiko Ichihara, talks about 'good time clubs,' which concretize Haruyama's concept of good time living.

> One of the most salient characteristics of our "good time clubs" is its aim to "let the old age shine" through various activities. It is of utmost importance that the residents get out of their rooms and socialize with others. They did not join us to live alone in their respective rooms. It is also sad if their pleasure consists only in looking at beautiful sceneries or living in a room that reminds one of an expensive hotel. What is more important is the way they conduct their activities in everyday life. So one can say that the activities of "good time clubs" are central to our concept of living in our assisted nursing home (my translation).

She explains that her first encounter with Haruyama's idea that the elderly must also enjoy their life as vigorously as possible was inspiring. Calling the residents 'guests' rather than 'residents,' she believes it is their job to 'do [their] very best' to help them realize 'the enjoyment of life.'

The club activities that are offered free of charge are watercolor painting, bingo games, *shamisen* playing, singing, *haiku* writing, calligraphy, meditation, gymnastics, Mahjong, and watching films. The activities that are offered at an extra cost are Hawaiian dance, karaoke, massages, flower arranging, gardening, art therapy, and nail and facial treatments and care. Various other events are regularly arranged, such as dancing and drinking parties, in which the staff participate together with the residents. The residents' relatives are invited, as well. The staff, the residents' relatives, and the old people mingle and dance together and enjoy a cup of sake and the music; this was mentioned as a representative event very much in the spirit of Haruyama's concept of *good time*. Exhibitions of the residents' art and craft works and concerts are held regularly. Sightseeing trips to hot springs, flower viewing tours, and so on are also arranged, often at an extra cost.

Another pillar in the strategies underlying Tsuru no sato's philosophy is the vigorous in-house training given to all staff from care workers, receptionist, and security guards to the workforce in the kitchen. All newcomers go through initial training, which lasts for about a month. Each month a seminar or a further training session consisting of two parts is arranged; one on manners and treatment of the guests, and the other on how to communicate with old people with dementia.

The staff are also encouraged to give residents (especially female residents) positive comments on their clothes, hairstyles, and accessories. In addition, the manager also tries to promote active interaction between the helpers and the guests, which sometimes creates unforeseeable problems. It is not uncommon that some of the guests, in old age, start behaving rather 'childishly.' For example, one guest aged seventy-four, Mrs B., developed a special attachment to one of the young, attentive male helpers, T. Mrs B. invited him to drink beer in her room in the evening, something he did on several occasions after he finished work (when he was off duty). Mrs B. subsequently started imagining that their relationship was very special. She bought him gifts, and would turn very sour if he attended to the needs of other guests on the same floor. Seeing the problem, the manager intervened, transferring him to another floor to lessen their daily contact. She made sure, however, that Mrs B. did not get the feeling that she was behaving improperly in any way (on the contrary, the manager gave her a signal that it was positive to be 'in love' at her age). The helper, T., returned all the gifts he received from Mrs B. to her relatives, who promised they would not tell Mrs B. Mrs B.'s 'crush' on T. subsided as their contact lessened.

The manager also takes pains to combat in a discreet manner the Japanese custom of giving gifts and souvenirs, something that may escalate into encouragement of partial treatment or even corruption. The guests are only allowed to give small amounts of sweets and snacks as a souvenir to the staff as a whole (not to any one person in particular). Everything else is returned to their relatives with a plea to keep quiet about it.

The manager clearly exercises authority to decide on irregular matters that concern the interaction between staff and guests. One can say that it is a rather hierarchical decision-making process, and the success of management depends very much on the character of the manager herself. She has been the general manager of the home since its opening in 2004, and as her profile in the *Misora* interview suggests, she was headhunted because of her previous position as the chief nurse in a local city hospital and her thirty years of experience as a registered nurse. Reiterating Haruyama's philosophy that their moral obligation is to do their very best for the guests, she emphasizes the importance of being flexible in accommodating the wishes of the residents. She tries to inculcate this positive and constructive attitude to the staff in order to make allowances for eventualities that may arise. If a guest comes up with a request that falls outside their ordinary work, their first reaction should be to see if there is room or leeway in their routines to accommodate the guest's wish.

As an example, she cites the case of seventy-four-year-old Mrs A., who loves to go shopping. She has Parkinson's disease, and is not allowed to go out alone because she has difficulty walking. Being more or less confined to the home, she has asked if she can get assistance once a month to go to a department store located in a nearby city. Needless to say, this is outside the care work that can be provided with the insurance money (which means she would have to pay the cost of attendance by a staff member from her own pocket). Besides, complying with her wish would require time from the staff. Nevertheless, the staff managed to solve the problem by finding a time slot and a willing staff who knows Mrs A. well, which made Mrs A. immensely happy.

When it comes to food, the most impressive aspect seen from a non-Japanese perspective is the care with which the meals are prepared. (As is well known, the Japanese preoccupation with food and nutrition is widespread across the class divisions, and I would assume the same can be said about institutions in the public sector as well.) Starting with breakfast in either Japanese or Western style, the staff serve warm meals three times a day, and a snack with tea or coffee at an extra cost. At an average cost of about 800 yen a meal, the meals are by no means exclusive, but the menu always includes two or three side dishes consisting mainly of vegetables of different colors in addition to the main dish. One can choose between two menus (or *a la carte* at an extra cost). At around three o'clock tea and coffee are served with homemade sweets (cheesecake, pumpkin pie, custard pudding, blueberry mousse, etc.) at the cost of 200 yen. The residents' guests can join them in dining at short notice, with an extra cost of about 1000 yen.[17]

This salient feature of Tsuru no sato—its hotel-like approach that treats residents more like guests, their *Miss Butlers*—seems at times to run counter to the principle of self-sufficiency. If a resident walks past one of the staff on the way to an elevator, for example, the staff hurries to the elevator to push the button, even if the resident is perfectly capable of doing it. The serving of a meal begins with a helper handing the residents warm hand towels. The helpers serve and clear the table for them when the meal is over. The manager has pointed out the strict training they receive in serving tea, coffee, and food, which includes detailed instruction regarding the placement of the rice bowl, soup bowl, the main dish, various side dishes, the glass, and chopsticks. The staff members also empty the rubbish bins, clean the residents' rooms, take their laundry, and come back with their clothes and towels neatly folded for them—again, regardless of the degree of their disability. (I have actually heard some of the residents complaining they would rather do the laundry and cleaning themselves.) From the point of view of self-sufficiency, it is problematic for one-third of the residents whose dependency is moderate, who should be encouraged to participate more in their everyday chores.[18] It also brings up the question of legitimizing an unfair distribution of social welfare that Kittay discussed in connection with Goodin's pragmatic ought. The management at Tsuru no sato seems to assume that it is more important to give the residents a feeling that they are treated like guests than to cultivate their spirit of independence.

In this connection, it is important to remember that most of the residents are middle-class women more than eighty years of age who were brought up in relatively wealthy homes in the 1920s and 1930s, when a class consciousness was much more apparent than today.[19] They also belong to a generation of housewives steeped in the hierarchical culture of the *ie* system, in which they were taught to dedicate themselves to the care of their 'demanding' old parents-in-law while young, and to look forward to old age when they could expect the same of the younger generation in return. This is the time when they should finally be allowed to be self-indulgent, and self-sufficiency is not necessarily on their priority list. Many of them would actually feel justified in being 'demanding' and do have a tendency to complain.

Many of the complaints I have overheard among the female residents have to do with the meals; that they serve radish too often; that noodles are served too cold; that the shellfish in the miso soup are not thoroughly washed; that the vegetables are overcooked and not crunchy; that no fresh vegetable is available for breakfast (Mrs Y.). They belong to a generation for whom serving overcooked vegetables to your aging mother-in-law who likes crunchy vegetables was a shame. Serving fresh vegetables on the breakfast table was a must if your father-in-law preferred it that way. By moving to Tsuru no sato, they had to acknowledge the fact that the wind of the time is not blowing their way anymore. Many of them therefore came to Tsuru no sato with a reluctant heart. Aware of this ambivalence in the minds of the residents, Tsuru no sato makes extended efforts to meet their demands.

For the sake of equal treatment, should one tell ninety-three year old Mrs Y., who has dutifully served her demanding parents-in-law in her younger days, to forget about her vegetables for breakfast? Should one tell Mrs A. to forget about her shopping? Or can one argue that making these options available might make sense from the perspective of the rationality of caring if it means much for their wellbeing? In the case of Tsuru no sato, they do it at an extra cost of 250 yen for Mrs Y., and 1700 yen an hour for Mrs A. Mrs

Y. was satisfied with her little bowl of salad in the morning, and seemed to think the price reasonable; Mrs A. was equally happy. The problem is not solved, however, for those who cannot afford to pay the extra expenses. This problem should not be forgotten, although it will not be discussed in the present chapter.

Browsing internet sites for private senior housing, one finds countless advertisements for private nursing homes in the Tokyo region, all of which try to compete for the prospective resident's attention. Besides common, overarching management concepts such as security and trust, eye-catching phrases such as 'healthy and tasty meals representing the best of the Japanese four seasons,' 'informal atmosphere,' 'the relatively low degree of dependence among the residents and freedom,' 'urban surroundings,' and 'affordable living expenses' decorate their home pages.[20] A couple of them advertise 'respect for self-sufficiency' as a motto, and one of the homes, Alive Care Home, states that depending on the condition of the residents, they may be asked to help set the dinner table for themselves, or fold their own laundry.[21] Compared to other private senior housing facilities, Tsuru no sato does seem to distinguish itself with its rather formal, hotel-like regime with its treatment of residents as Mrs Butlers.[22] Despite the differences in the areas of focus, however, there seems to be a common tendency among private care homes to advertise their readiness to cater to the special needs of their target group. In other words, the profiles of the target group may vary, but the advertisers all emphasize their flexible responsiveness to individual client needs. In that sense, Tsuru no sato can also be said to be representative. It remains to be seen, however, whether or not the private care homes can all live up to their mottoes in reality to the same reasonable degree as Tsuru no sato seems to do.

The contrast is striking when one looks at the more or less standardized homepages of the Norwegian nursing homes listed under each municipality. It is no doubt partly because the standard of housing and the quality of care is presumed to be relatively even and reasonably high, and the net expenses (adjusted according to the income of the residents) are more or less the same regardless of whether a home is run by a municipality or by a private company on consignment. It is, however, also partly because there is currently such a long waiting list for entry into a nursing home that one often cannot afford to be selective anyway. The evaluation of the clients' physical and mental conditions to allow acceptance into a nursing home is undertaken by a committee made up of doctors and other health professionals in each municipality. Many municipalities in the 1990s introduced a WHO-inspired principle that emphasizes the importance of providing health care in the patients' homes rather than at institutions.[23] In accordance with this principle, delaying their move to an institution by giving as much home help as possible was thought to benefit both the elderly and the municipalities, because it was more cost effective than building nursing homes. As Karla Larsen, a district nurse at the home help station in Oslo, told me, the threshold for being accepted into a nursing home was much higher in 2008 than in the 1990s. She says that 'equal accessibility'[24] of help and self-sufficiency are the principles of care most taken for granted in the Norwegian system. The home help services are free of charge and are available for every resident in need of health care at home, regardless of citizenship. Their motto is to help the elderly to be self-sufficient and to live at home as long as possible. They are therefore cautious about giving more help than is needed. As a rule of the thumb, they would consider sending someone to a nursing home first when home help service is needed more than twelve times a day (one visit can be as short as fifteen minutes), which means the person needs assistance in connection with most basic, everyday chores. It is only when one has dementia that one would be given priority regardless of physical dependency.

Once accepted into a nursing home, one is likely to be satisfied as far as the material standards are concerned. The care homes that I have observed in the Oslo region are divided into relatively small units of eight to ten residents (Tsuru no sato has twenty-nine residents on each floor, which forms a unit), each equipped with its own kitchen/dining room and a living space. Efforts to make the living quarters look like *home* are evident.[25] The individual rooms are spacious, and the kitchen area has a big dining table where residents can sit and talk with care workers over coffee. The emphasis on the home-like atmosphere is reflected in the informal and casual way of address and association among the care workers and the dependents. Cultural activities are arranged for special celebratory occasions such as Christmas, New Year, and the National Day, but there are very few organized daily activities of the sort offered at Japanese nursing homes. This is because most residents would feel more at ease socializing with other residents and care workers in a 'natural' atmosphere, I was told. One helper told me that many residents were simply not up to any organized activities because of their physical conditions, a comment that implies, however, that some residents actually are capable. It is not unthinkable that some might in fact appreciate more activities to break the monotony of everyday life.[26]

The care workers bring food to the table, and the residents who can, make their own open sandwiches and help themselves to coffee or tea. A warm meal is served once a day. Most other everyday chores are done by the care workers, not because the residents are treated as guests, but because their dependency level is high. One eighty-three-year-old female resident told me she was lucky to be there, and that she felt almost bad about having lived there for as long as five years (the average time an elderly person spends in a nursing home is two years), implying that she is sorry to occupy a place that someone else could have.[27]

Life experiences and the expectations of residents in Norwegian nursing homes are naturally different from their counterparts in Japan, or in most other countries. Two of the nursing homes I visited were located in city wards with relatively high immigrant populations, but there was only one elderly resident with a Pakistani background in one home and no immigrants in the other. I was told that most Asian and African immigrants would avoid placing their elderly in nursing homes because they would feel alienated in such a 'culturally Norwegian environment.'[28] I have also talked to a Japanese immigrant husband who has refused to send his aging wife with Alzheimer's disease to a nursing home because he 'cannot possibly let her eat milk porridge for dinner on Saturday.'[29] There is little room for individual adjustments of services, even at extra cost in a Norwegian nursing home—regardless of whether it is private or public—unless the adjustments are related to health care. As the elderly immigrant population grows, the need to take their special life situations into consideration must be taken seriously. As already noted, feminist scholars have problematized the standardized concept of care in public management, and have called for a less bureaucratic system that allows room for flexibility to accommodate 'the individual and the particular,' which is so vital in a care-giving relationship. It remains to be seen whether or not they will succeed in combating the problem of rigidity in the highly bureaucratized system without letting more market forces intervene.[30]

It should be noted here, however, that the purpose of this comparison is not to argue for the supremacy of one system over the other. Regardless of whether one is dealing with private or public institutions in the Japanese LTCI System or in the tax-based Nordic system, what matters in the end is the quality of care seen in the light of the dependent's relative position. Let us remind ourselves once again of Kittay's statement that the question of equality fragments into questions of equalities: 'Equality *for whom*? Equality *by what measure*? Equality *of what*? Equal *to whom*?' (Kittay 1999: 5). Moving away from the classical liberalist notion of equality, which presupposes that all members of society are independent, *rational* beings, towards a more connection-based notion of equality that accommodates the inevitable variety of human interactions will necessarily involve making corresponding adjustments in the assessment of the legitimacy of vulnerability claims. The notions of equality and self-sufficiency need to be relativized in terms not only of the particular relationship between the caregiver and care receiver, but also in terms of the care receiver's earlier connections, his/her life experiences.

This is not to say that the caregiver must necessarily accept all the vulnerability claims, but he or she must carefully take the various factors influencing the situation of the care receiver into consideration. The connection-based care work that accommodates the inevitable variety of human interactions presupposes a considerable degree of intimacy between the caregiver and her/his dependent and a familiarity with the care recipient's life and circumstances. Senior housing facilities have a potential advantage over home services in that they can provide greater opportunities to build more solid relations of care because of the longer hours of interaction between the staff and the residents—stronger relations of care that should, in turn, make it easier for the staff to assess the nature of their obligation in that particular relationship with *rational* flexibility.

Conclusion

There have been many critical comments about the LTCI in Japan, especially from an academia that prefers to see the Japanese welfare system develop more in the direction of the Nordic model of public welfare system with the standardized, equal treatment of everyone, regardless of their economic standing and place of residence.[31] Transferring one system of care that functions reasonably well in one culture to another culture with a different socio-historical background is not necessarily easy, however. Pointing out the Japanese people's fundamental lack of trust in the government as a major obstacle in developing Nordic-style public welfare in Japan and dismissing its possibility, Chizuko Ueno urges us instead to appreciate what the 2000 LTCI has done, rather than what it has not done. In response to criticism that its benefits have been unevenly distributed, she argues that the LTCI has achieved the political goal of 'alleviating the burden of the care in the middle income class,' as originally planned. If it did not do the same for those with low incomes, we should strive to 'implement another set of remedies to help the lower income class in the future' (Ueno 2007: 178).

Its achievement also needs to be seen in the Japanese historical context. As already noted, the welfare of the elderly in Japan was long based on the premise that women in the family were morally obligated to bear the burden of dependency care. It was considered shameful for the family to commit its elderly to institutional care. The aged parents would, in return, do their utmost to bequeath their assets to their children, feeling guilty about using money for their own leisure and pleasure. The joy of life in old age was supposed to come from this mutual dependence, which has been a vital cornerstone in supporting family values in Japan.

Many women have persevered in their traditional role, but have been bitterly disappointed to see their own daughters and daughters-in-law refusing to live up to expectation. Many of the dutiful women have had the bitter experience of seeing male siblings who did not participate in the care of the parents assuming equal rights to inheritance. The synergic intergenerational relationship based on mutual dependence, which used to settle the plus and minus accounts nicely in the old *ie* system, does not seem to be working.[32] In order to stop the vicious circle of betrayed expectations, it is of decisive importance to subvert the image of the elderly as frugal but demanding people who expect their children to sacrifice freedom for their sake. The LTCI and an institution such as Tsuru no sato have done their share to change this image of old people. As banal as it may sound to the Western ear, the notion of good time living can be considered epoch making in this context.

As Nancy Fraser, an American political scientist, points out, the focus on the problem of justice in social and cultural politics has shifted from *redistribution* to *recognition* in the post-1989, post-socialist age. People now fight for the recognition of socially or culturally oppressed groups, rather than the redistribution of wealth, which was a key concept when people still believed in socialism. Arguing that we need both, Fraser warns us not to overemphasize the former at the expense of the latter, or vice versa. What is important in this context is that she reminds us that a term of group differentiation such as 'gender' and 'the elderly' is 'not only a political-economic differentiation but a cultural-valuational differentiation as well:' the images of group differentiation cannot be corrected by 'political-economic redistribution alone but require additional independent remedies of recognition' (Fraser 1997: 20). The LTCI and a new way of thinking such as Haruyama's good time living have contributed to giving a much needed positive (and different) cultural-valuational differentiation to the elderly as an independent group in Japan. Recognizing their claim for their new identity is tantamount to recognizing the corresponding claim of the women who would have been their caregivers within the households. It is first by taking care of the needs of the elderly that one can start thinking about the needs of their daughters, real or in-law, and liberate them from the traditional burden of care. In other words, a need to familiarize and popularize a new concept of the old age has been more acute in Japan than in other countries where there is a more equal distribution of dependency work. By helping to establish a national consensus that 'the care of the elderly is no longer just the family obligation,' the LTCI was no less than a 'family revolution,' if I am to borrow Chizuko Ueno's words again (Ueno 2007: 177–8).[33]

This is not to say, however, that the reform poses no problems. Excessive emphasis on market-friendly values might cultivate the *false* needs of the dependents at the expense of other important needs of the elderly, such as self-sufficiency and self-reliance. One may argue that the thinking behind the hotel-like service found in Tsuru no sato falls under this category. There is no doubt that the major challenge for private institutions such as Tsuru no sato (and many other facilities that profile themselves as providing services, to varying degrees, on the client's terms) lies in finding the right balance between offering good dependency work and supporting self-sufficiency. As the terms and conditions of the LTCI will predictably get tougher in the future due to lack of funding, private nursing homes will have to find ways to make ends meet. Hopefully they will solve financial problems by encouraging residents to learn to do more things on their own, rather than by giving even more services and charging more fees.[34]

Finally, going back to Kittay's proposal, I would like to conclude by arguing that 'what is required is an appreciation of the inevitable variety of human interactions' and life situations. In this context, one can perhaps argue that the greatest achievement of the LTCI is that it has encouraged institutions of various origin, status, and size, from private entrepreneurs and cooperatives to NPOs, NGOs, and social foundations, to establish care businesses with distinct marketing profiles, thereby making it easier for people of different economical and cultural standing to find what suits their specific needs best.

Chizuko Ueno, among others, has been an exponent for welfare pluralism, even as she makes it clear that she favors cooperatives, since she believes that cooperatives can, to a much larger extent than private enterprises, work out the details of individual care plans in close consultation with the care recipients and their families, and are positioned to encourage self-sufficiency of the care recipients. She sees them positively as one of the best and most viable alternatives, while at the same time endorsing the present system that keeps a variety of options open to others in different life situations (Ueno 2007: 184).

Depending on the inevitable variety of life situations surrounding the care recipients, some may find it easier to solve their problems in private senior housing (senior apartments and nursing homes) with good facilities, whereas others may seek their solutions in small-scale nursing homes with more modest profiles, while most will opt to stay home by combining the benefits of the LTCI and help from their family members. If the public (state) can do its job of maintaining the availability of various alternatives and options to everyone at reasonable cost, the prospect of such a *multi-faceted welfare society* may not be a utopian dream. We can at least begin to foresee the possibility of such a scenario, even as we know there are obstacles.

Chapter 5
The Work Situations of Home Helpers in Japan and Norway

Unni Edvardsen

Home helpers constitute an essential element within elderly care—helping the elderly with practical tasks and enabling them to continue living at home. Yet, there is little knowledge about the daily professional challenges that home helpers face and little awareness in the public of the important role they play in society. The present study attempts to rectify this imbalance by focusing on home helpers' work and work conditions in Japan and Norway, two countries with different elderly care traditions.

Home helpers constitute one of several professional groups within elderly care, and the relationship is characterized by the recipient's dependence on help and the home helper's obligation to provide help that the recipient needs and is entitled to.[1] Consequently, I try to relate the empirical findings to the theoretical concepts of structural and relational power in care relationships, discussing the likely effect of structural conditions on relational power.

The structure of this chapter is as follows. First, perspectives on care and care relationships are discussed. Then, in the main part of this chapter, findings from a study on home helpers and their work situations in Japan and Norway are presented. Last, I sum up the findings and discuss these in the light of the theoretical perspectives of relational and structural power.

Theoretical foundation: the concepts of care and relational power

Home helper work tasks consist of household chores such as cleaning and preparing meals for recipients. In other words, we are talking about help with physical tasks that recipients can no longer manage on their own. However, home help also involves aspects of social and psychological wellbeing. As such home help is both a social service (practical help) and care.[2] According to Martinsen (in Gough 1987), care consists of three components: a social relation, an understanding for the other, and an attitude that recognizes the recipient in his/her situation. This kind of relationship is fostered by experiencing situations with the recipient, and seeing how the recipient relates to his/her own situation.

A care relationship entails emotional involvement and responsibility. To acquire an understanding of the other takes time, as it is a question of trust that develops over time. Compared to this, care *service* is more like a commodity, not demanding the same degree of involvement from the helper. Services are more standardized, with less individual adaptation.

It is an underlying assumption of this chapter that organizational and other structural conditions have an impact on care and the relationship between the home helper and user. One may look upon this as a dilemma between what is possible for the helper to do within the scope of structural conditions and what is needed for a care relationship.

In the following I take Karen Christensen's model of analyzing the development of home care services as a stepping stone to develop my own theoretical underpinnings for the present study. Christensen distinguishes between structural and relational power (Christensen 2005). Structural power can be ideological, legal, organizational, or economic. Relational power is visible in people's interactions and 'is characterized by the kind of relation those actors actually have at any one time' (Christensen 2005: 34). Between these she makes room for an intermediate position for reflections and value orientation, which give direction to care interactions. Characteristic of this intermediate position is the concept of the rationality of caring, which she connects to *other orientation*, a dialogue within care giving that aims to strengthen individuality and self-determination in the recipient. As a precondition for other orientation to take place, the caregiver must have a certain level of freedom of action and a certain level of power. Christensen distinguishes between three phases of development of home care services, each roughly corresponding to the decades of the 1970s to 1990s. She finds that structural power has become more explicit, controlling increasingly more of the relational space, thereby reducing care relational power to occasional opportunities at the individual level.

In the present analysis, the concept of relational power is to be linked even more strongly to Martinsen's concept of care. It is understood as the ability (1) to be affected, in the sense of being open, sensitive, and empathic, and (2) to affect or influence others by the way one has been influenced by and responds to the other. The opposite of relational power is unilateral power—when one person increases his or her ability to affect the other while remaining unaffected by the other (Mesle 1983). Since care relationships are asymmetric in terms of formal and symbolic power, it is easy to envisage the latter scenario.

Christensen's concept of the intermediate position is in the current analysis filled by the home helper. Structures constitute the framework for relational power and set limits for the home helper's interactions with the recipient.[3] Since care entails that the home helper acts and thinks in the interest of the recipient, knowing the recipient and having the ability to empathize are vital preconditions for care rationality (Gough 1987; Wærness 1999). As developing trust and getting to know the recipient take time, it is important that there is enough time for each visit (without having to rush), and that there is regularity in terms of having the same helper(s) visit the recipient over a longer period of time.

In analyzing the empirical data in the next part, I look at different structural conditions for home helpers' work and discuss their likely impacts on relational power.

Empirical analysis

The empirical analysis has two sources of primary data: interviews and a survey (questionnaire).[4] A total of fifty-four interviews were conducted with home helpers, elderly recipients, and managers in both Japan and Norway, using the same interview guides in both countries. Data was collected in 2005 and 2006.[5]

The survey of home helpers consisted of about fifty questions. It was distributed to home helpers in both countries. Altogether, 366 questionnaires have been analyzed, using the statistical software SPSS—163 from Japan and 203 from Norway. In addition to the questions that could be coded and analyzed in SPSS, the questionnaire had six open questions and some fields open for comments.

In the following I focus on various structural aspects of home helpers' work in Japan and Norway, discussing their significance for relational power. I look at background characteristics of helpers, work load, content of work, amount of help for users, stability of the user–helper relationship, and organization of work and work conditions.

Helper characteristics

The mean age of the Japanese home helpers in the current study was fifty-one, ranging from the youngest at twenty to the eldest at seventy-one. In Norway the mean age was forty-eight, ranging from nineteen to sixty-eight years.[6] Looking at age segments, the largest segment of helpers were in their fifties in both countries.

Does it matter to elderly recipients how old the home helpers are? Some elderly say they don't have much in common to talk about with young people. One said he felt comfortable in conversation with his helpers who were in their fifties and sixties (implying that he did not feel so comfortable talking with younger helpers). Also, other studies indicate that users may feel insecure when the home helper is quite young (Elster 1995). Older helpers may have a different value orientation than younger ones, and presumably are more understanding of their life stories. They also have more experience in terms of practical tasks such as cooking. On the other hand, how well a helper and recipient get along together is also a matter of chemistry between two personalities. Moreover, helpers in their sixties are physically weaker than younger helpers. This could cause problems in cases of bedridden elderly, when there is a need to lift recipients.

Above we saw that the mean age of home helpers is about three years higher in Japan than in Norway. Does this also mean that they have worked longer within elderly care? Not if we judge by the survey results. The mean number of years of experience within elderly care was eight years in Japan and eleven in Norway. Moreover, one-quarter of helpers in Norway have worked for more than twenty years within elderly care; only 5% of the Japanese helpers have such long experience. This finding indicates that in Japan women tend to start working professionally later in life, often staying at home while their children are young. In Norway women are employees even when their children are young.

Work load

Many home helpers in both countries work part time. According to the survey, 71% of Japanese home helpers work part time compared to 53% in Norway. These figures are very high, but were expected. According to the survey, Norwegian home helpers work thirty-one hours per week, and Japanese home helpers work twenty hours. Given the fact that Japanese home helpers work more than ten hours less per week than their counterparts in Norway, it is expected that the work load in terms of number of recipients is significantly less, and in fact the number of recipients (per helper) is less than half in Japan (see Table 5.1). This can also be related to the length of each visit. The questionnaire asked how often a home helper was at a recipient's house for less than thirty minutes and more than ninety minutes. Given the significantly smaller number of recipients that home helpers have in Japan, it is expected that it is more common to stay longer. According to the survey, more than 90% of the Japanese home helpers stay for more than one-and-a-half hours at the recipient's home once or several times per week. The figure for Norway is 73%.

The total number of recipients per home helper in Japan is just three more than the number they visit per week. Thus it is reasonable to conclude that

Table 5.1: Work load

	Japan	Norway
Mean working hours per week	20	31
Mean number of recipients per week	9	25
Mean number of recipients in ordinary day	2.7	6.6
Mean number of recipients in total	12	50

(N = 352)

they visit most of their recipients once every week. The total number of recipients for Norwegian helpers appears very large (fifty). This is related to the factors mentioned above, as well as to two other elements. In a few municipalities helpers work in teams of two, thereby covering twice as many recipients during a day/week. However, home helpers in most municipalities in Norway work alone, not in teams. Working full time and alone, they manage to clean in the homes of about five recipients a day. The second factor contributing to the large number of recipients per helper in Norway is that recipients in Norway seem to get practical help more seldom than recipients in Japan. I will return to this issue below.

If we look at the conditions for relational power based on the findings above, it is quite clear that the work situation for home helpers in Japan is more amicable. Japanese home helpers have few recipients, so they are able to get to know them all. As for Norway, the situation is more like an assembly line model (cf. Szebehely 1995). It is unlikely that helpers have time or interest in trying to get to know all the recipients they visit. In the survey, the helpers were asked in how many instances they knew the recipients' main life stories. The results confirm the assumptions. Of the Japanese home helpers, 58% knew the life stories of *all* their recipients, compared to only 11% in Norway, and 85% of the home helpers in Japan knew the life stories of *more than half* the recipients. The corresponding figure for Norway was 48%. The main reason for this gap probably is to be found in the frequency with which home helpers visit recipients, the length of the visits, and the number of recipients per helper. In Norway the number of recipients for each home helper is greater and they visit each recipient more seldom. Most people don't share personal information with people that they only see once in a while. It takes time to build trust in a relationship. One Norwegian home helper said, 'I notice that the more often I go there, the more they appreciate it when I come, and each time they open up more.'

With structural conditions as described above in terms of work load, the space for *other orientation* and relational power seems smaller in Norway than in Japan. Also, other studies have pointed out that the number of recipients, the length of each visit, and whether they have regular recipients has an impact on how well the home helper gets to know recipients and on the quality of care (Næss and Wærness 1996).

Content of work

The main task of home helpers is to do the daily housework chores. How often home helpers do different tasks for their recipients is related to several factors—the way services are organized, including how tasks are assigned to different professions, and the tasks that are not included in the elderly care provision system in each country.[7]

The data from the questionnaire suggests that Norwegian home helpers clean more than home helpers in Japan. Of the Norwegian helpers, 74% said they clean daily, compared to 41% in Japan. On the other hand, home helpers in Japan seem to do a greater variety of tasks for/with the recipients, such as going shopping for the recipient, making lunch or dinner, washing clothes for recipients, or helping recipients take a bath (see the appendix at the end of this chapter). The chore with the greatest difference between helpers in the two countries is making lunch or dinner for recipients. While 80% of Japanese helpers do this weekly, only 36% of the Norwegian helpers do it this often, and more than half of them never do it. The only tasks in the survey that the Norwegian home helpers do more often than the helpers in Japan, apart from cleaning, are having a cup of tea/coffee with recipients and making the recipients' beds.[8]

The list of tasks that home helpers never do (Table 5.2) also makes quite interesting reading. There are four tasks that more than half of the home helpers in Norway never do: accompanying recipients on a walk or to shop, accompanying them to medical doctors, making lunch or dinner for recipients, and helping recipients with bathing. In Japan there is only one item among the tasks in Table 5.2 that more than half of the home helpers never do, namely having a cup of coffee or tea with the recipient. Since having a cup of tea/coffee with the recipient is not included as a public service in either country, the score on this was low for both countries, but probably for different reasons. In Japan it is prohibited for the helper to have a cup of tea/coffee with recipients; in Norway it may not be forbidden, but, as the time designated for different chores is barely enough to complete the work, there is no time to sit down for five minutes after finishing the

Table 5.2: Tasks that home helpers never do (%)

	Japan	Norway
Accompany recipient on a walk or to shop	38.7	74.4
Have a cup of coffee/tea with the recipient	68.5	23.0
Accompany recipient to medical doctor	33.8	63.6
Make lunch or dinner for recipient	14.3	52.3
Help with bathing	34.6	52.0

(N = 346–355)

cleaning in the recipient's house. If they do, they will be late for the next recipient.

It is hard to tell what content of work configuration constitutes the best conditions for relational power—whether more cleaning tasks or more varied tasks foster more conversation and understanding. Instantly one may think it is the ones with the more varied tasks; however, going shopping for the recipient, as many Japanese helpers do, entails being away from the recipient quite a lot. On the other hand, it is hard to hold a conversation while vacuum cleaning or cleaning the bathroom. The two activities with the greatest potential for social interaction—having a cup of coffee/tea and accompanying recipients on a walk or to shop—are at the top of the 'never do' list in Japan and Norway respectively. It may be easy to blame home helpers for failing to do these things, but even though home helpers are often considered social contacts for recipients, social care is simply not covered through the system of home help services in either of the countries.

The home helpers in the survey were asked if there were any task(s) that they would like to have more time for. Exactly the two things that they do least were mentioned, namely (1) to accompany the recipient for a walk or to shop, and (2) to be a conversation partner (i.e. to have time to sit down for a chat and listen to the recipient). Many helpers underscored how important this is in order to cheer up the recipients and give them more motivation and interest in living. Also, doing things together with recipients, such as cleaning or making meals, were mentioned; however, the respondents noted that the time designated for the visits is too short to allow for involving the recipient. This is a paradox, since the policy of the governments in both Japan and Norway is to make able recipients more self-sufficient, preventing them from deteriorating in health and their *Activities of Daily Living* level. With the purpose of giving help being only to *assist* the recipient, the designated time for help is shortened, but, in fact, *assisting* the recipient may take longer than if the helper had just done it *for* the recipient.

Amount of help

Do elderly recipients of home help services get enough help? Of the Norwegian helpers, 82% said that they thought some of the recipients they go to are in need of *more* help, compared to 59% in Japan. This may indicate that the time that elderly people get for home help often is too limited in Norway. The standard help for cleaning in many municipalities in Norway now is one to two hours (depending on the size of house, etc.) every two or three weeks. If the recipient has special needs (e.g. due to a health problem that makes the recipient soil the flat very often), the regularity of visits by home helpers will increase, but the time for each visit is shortened. In Japan recipients, even in care level 1, can receive home help services several times/ hours a week. In Japan there is a user fee of 10% on all kinds of Long-Term Care Insurance services. In Norway home visiting nursing services are free (including help with bathing), but recipients have to pay per hour for help with housework (the municipalities set the price per hour, usually in steps depending on income).

Several of the Norwegian home helpers I interviewed said that they think that many elderly do not get help *often* enough and that the time designated for each chore in the care plan in many instances is a bit too short. Given the fact that the physical and mental conditions of elderly recipients vary from day to day, some tasks may take longer on 'bad days.' For example, if the home helper is to assist a demented person with dressing, it may take half an hour just to persuade the person to agree to do it. The time for tackling such unpredictable occurrences is not included in the care plan time budget and, as such, is not included in the home helpers' working hours.[9]

Related to this is the question of whether home helpers often see that recipients have needs that are insufficiently covered, and what these needs are. Table 5.3 shows that the top two needs are the same in both countries. An overwhelming majority of the helpers in Norway and close to half of the helpers in Japan consider social contact/conversation and accompanying recipients on walks as the two uncovered needs that they see most often among elderly recipients. Nearly 90% of the Norwegian home helpers consider lack of social contact/conversation as an uncovered need among elderly recipients. Many helpers in both countries mentioned how difficult it is to leave lonely recipients, and some even mentioned that they stay a bit longer if they can. Table 6.3 also shows that a much greater proportion of the

Table 5.3: Percentage of home helpers who see unmet needs among elderly recipients (sorted after the Japanese 'scores')

Unmet need	Japan	Norway
Accompany for walk	47	72
Social contact/conversation	47	87
Information re services, rights, etc.	44	44
Tidying up	28	66
Security	20	45
Technical equipment	19	27
Making meals	18	39
Washing clothes	18	49
Personal care	15	38
Shopping/errand	9	50
Cleaning	6	38

(N = 366)

home helpers in Norway often see uncovered needs among elderly recipients than their colleagues in Japan. This could have to do with higher expectations among Norwegian helpers, and the level and kind of help they think elderly *ought* to get. But it can also be explained in line with the finding above that Japanese elderly recipients of home help services actually get more help than elderly in Norway.

Related to the question of whether elderly recipients of home care get enough help or not is the question as to whether recipients ask their home helpers to do things that are not in the care plan/contract. Of the Norwegian helpers, 40% answered that this happens weekly, compared to 12% in Japan. There may be several factors contributing to this large difference between the two countries. One is that the system may be stricter in Japan regarding what home helpers are allowed by their employers to do. In Norway a home helper is generally allowed to do things outside the care plan for a recipient if the recipient asks for it and on the conditions that it is done within the time designated for the recipient and that the recipient is willing to compromise on the time for tasks in the care plan (e.g. the helper cleans the refrigerator instead of cleaning the floor). A second factor is that Japanese recipients know that they are not entitled to get any other help and thus do not ask for it. One recipient said, 'I know what they can do and cannot, according to their job description. For example, they are not supposed to clean up the backyard. I try not to ask them to do what they should not do.' A helper said, 'We have to ask for permission from the office for any deviation from the plan.' I also asked whether the home helpers do, in fact, do work outside the care plan when asked by the recipients. Of the Norwegian home helpers, 30% said that they do so weekly, compared to 8% in Japan.

The findings described above indicate that elderly recipients in Norway get less help and have more uncovered needs than elderly recipients in Japan.[10] And when the time designated for the practical chores is a bit short, it may even be hard to treat the recipient with due dignity and respect, as it often takes more time to do things in dialogue with fragile, vulnerable, and maybe confused recipients. On the other hand, home helpers in Norway appear to be more flexible in terms of being willing to do other things than what the care plan says if the recipients ask. So, even when formal organizational structures give little room for care rationality and relational power, home helpers seem to use their intermediate position to slacken off on formal structures and to accommodate the recipients individually. Interview data shows that the managers condone this practice, provided it is within the designated time for the recipient and that he/she is willing to compromise on chores in the care plan for which the helper may not get time.

Stability of user–helper relationships

We know from a number of studies that it matters a lot to many elderly recipients that the same home helper (or just a few helpers) visits regularly (Næss and Wærness 1996; Rønning 2004; Szebehely 2003). This was also emphasized by the recipients who I interviewed in both Japan and Norway.

If the same helpers come for a longer period of time, they get to know the recipient's home, where things are, and how the recipient wants to have things done. One recipient put it this way: 'The best is to have someone that is used to me. They know how I am and how I want it.' Another one explained:

> Sometimes my helpers get sick and cannot come. The office offers a substitute, but I turn it down. With a totally unfamiliar face, I cannot have a chat, and I have to give her instructions from scratch. You know—where the dust cloth is and things like that. So whenever my [regular] helpers cannot come, the schedule is not filled (Japanese recipient, ninety-two).

Public helpers in Japan rotate every three to five years. Getting new helpers can make the recipient feel insecure and worry. Mr Suzuki has four different helpers who visit him. It has been the same for three years, but from April he will get new ones. When I spoke to him, he said that 'this is the problem that bothers me most. They are new in this neighborhood, and don't know where to get what, where the store is etc.'

Asked if they know who (which helper) is coming to help on a particular day, most Japanese recipients seem to know this. Helpers are assigned to particular recipients. Sickness and sick leave are exceptions when there may be unknown helpers who make the visit. In Norway this is often not the case. When recipients get cleaning only once every two or three weeks, then who is coming depends on the personnel rotation at the municipal domiciliary care service station. In this respect, the situation seemed better with private provider firms in Oslo. Managers I interviewed in the private provider firms said that they know how important this is to elderly recipients and thus try to designate specific helpers to recipients.

Organization and work conditions

What is everyday work life like for home helpers in Japan and Norway, and in what way can the daily routines and work conditions influence the space for relational power? In the following I look at schedules, travel to recipients, contact with colleagues, who to seek advice from, salary, and whether recipients have the same home helper(s) over time.

Schedule

Most people like to know when to expect visitors. This gives us a feeling of security and enables us to prepare for the visit and to make plans for the rest of the day. This study indicates that recipients of home care in Japan have the most predictable schedule. Table 6.4 shows that home helpers in Japan work according to exact schedules and that the recipients know exactly when to expect the helpers to come. One Japanese recipient who I interviewed said about the home helpers, 'they are as accurate as a clock. I sometimes think they are waiting right outside the door until the scheduled time.' In Norway a typical situation would be that at a morning meeting the helpers get a list of recipients they are to visit on that day. Then the helpers work through the list, calling at the homes of early risers first. It is not uncommon that they get calls for additional visits because someone is sick.

Travel to recipients and time between user appointments

Time spent on travel to recipients and waiting time between home care visits have an impact on the efficiency of the provider organization, and affect cost and work conditions and the efficiency of the individual home helper. Long waiting and/or travel hours are exhausting in the long run and may have a

Table 5.4: 'Is there normally an exact time set for when you are to call at recipients?'

	Japan	Norway
Yes, it is (e.g. 9.30)	96.9	21.6
Not exactly, but roughly (e.g. between 9.00 and 10.00)	3.1	43.8
Calling time given as morning, afternoon, etc.	0	13.9
It varies	0	20.6

(N = 354)

bad health effect on the employee, which in turn may have consequences for the clients. Private and public providers seem to have different practices. Having regular employees, public providers will always try to fill a home helper's schedule with as much user time as possible. However, for providers that mainly have part-time employees who get paid by the hour for each client, waiting and travel time does not matter economically, and hence is more common.

The survey asked for average time spent on travel from a helper's own home or office to recipients. The result was identical for both countries: 90% of home helpers spend less than thirty minutes travelling to recipients. In Japan home helpers mainly go to recipients who live in the vicinity where they themselves live, reducing time spent on travel. In Norway travel time is kept low by using cars.

In Japan, where most home helpers are not regular part-time employees, there is often waiting time between clients. For example, one helper who I interviewed worked for a private for-profit company Monday to Friday, and left home at seven o'clock every morning. However, in the morning he only worked for one hour, then he had to wait for his next visit at ten o'clock. The day I met him, he had finished at the home of one user at noon, but his next appointment was not until three o'clock. In the breaks he spent time in cafes, drinking tea. So, in fact, he had extra expenses due to the waiting time, but no income for these hours.

Home helpers' contact with colleagues

Qualification and payment indicates that being a home helper is a profession. Further characteristic of a profession are a certain level of professional consciousness and exchange of thoughts related to the job. Interviews indicate that home helpers in Japan in general (apart from public employees) go directly from their own homes to the users' homes, not seeing colleagues at all during a normal work day. Norwegian helpers are mainly employed by the municipality. They typically participate at a morning briefing, often with other care professionals, where they are informed about any changes regarding users (their state of being, new users, etc.). They may also be asked to step in for a colleague in the case of sickness.

In the survey, I looked at two kinds of activities that potentially foster collegial fellowship and that might be a source of help, sharing, and support, namely meetings and lunches with colleagues. I also asked whom home helpers first turn to if they have problems with recipients.

Lunch: a great majority of the Norwegian helpers (74%), compared to 19% of Japanese helpers, have lunch in a lunch room or canteen at the employer's office/home help station. Most Japanese home helpers have lunch at home (27.5%), while around 22% say that it varies.

Meetings: 83% of home helpers in both Japan and Norway participate in meetings regularly, either with other helpers or together with other care professions such as nurses. But, while nearly 100% of the Norwegian home helpers participate during work hours, less than half (42.6%) of the time spent at meetings by Japanese helpers is within work hours. Japanese meetings for home helpers may be in thc form of a *kenkyuukai*, a kind of study meeting. The problem is that such meetings are often held at weekends, when helpers would rather be with family; some don't receive any pay for participating.

Primary confidante: the questionnaire asked who the home helpers seek advice/help/support from if they have problems with recipients. The results were very similar for Japan and Norway. A great majority of home helpers in both countries (87%) first and foremost seek help/advice from the nearest leader at work. Colleagues come second, with 54% in both countries.

The findings above suggest that there is a big difference in terms of work environment and contact with colleagues between Japanese and Norwegian home helpers. Home helpers who have little contact with colleagues may, in the long run, feel lonely in their work. Without the chance to talk and discuss daily joys and problems, helpers may not get the refill of energy, collegial support, and professional reflection that is necessary in order to be a care rational home helper.

Salary

The salary for home helpers varies depending on experience and level of qualification. However, this study indicates that home helpers in Norway earn about twice as much as their colleagues in Japan. While the salary in Japan is 1200–1400 yen per hour, it is about 2380 yen (111 Norwegian krone) in Norway.[11] However, comparing salaries cross-nationally may not always make sense without taking various other factors into consideration. Among others, taxes are higher and food is more expensive in Norway than in Japan.

Moreover, apart from a small number who are publicly employed, home helpers in Japan get paid by the hour for the designated time with the recipients. They receive nothing for travel time and inconvenient waiting time between jobs (recipients). This contributes towards making the job of home helper as one of low status.

Discussion

This study has shown that Japanese and Norwegian home helpers share some common characteristics and challenges, but that their work conditions are quite different.

Home helpers in both countries seem to enjoy their work, mainly due to the important role that they feel they play in the lives of recipients. They expressed appreciation for having the chance to get to know elderly people who are rich in life experience, and said they can learn and grow as human beings. They also felt good about sensing the gratitude of recipients.

The nature of the home helpers' work is the same in Japan and Norway, though Norwegian helpers do more cleaning. Norwegian home helpers also have a greater work load in terms of number of recipients and working hours. With more time pressure between jobs and shorter time for each user, the feeling of stress is more common among Norwegian home helpers than it is in Japan. It is reasonable to believe that in Norway structural power is more explicit, giving less space for relational power. In Japan structures relating to this seem to allow for a larger space for relational power (at least prior to the implementation of the LTCI revision in April 2006).

On the other hand, when it comes to contact with colleagues and salary, work conditions for Japanese helpers may contribute towards less job satisfaction, which in turn may contribute towards less motivation to exert relational power. However, our findings do not support this assumption.

Still, home helpers in Japan and Norway face the same challenge: in order to enable private companies to be service providers within elderly care, services have become split into details (itemized), there is little time for doing the designated practical tasks, and there is no longer/very little time to have a chat with recipients. In other words, structural power has become more pronounced in both countries and work has become more stressful. This has made it more difficult to cultivate the psychological and emotional aspects of care, thereby reducing the sense of satisfaction among recipients, and the sense of meaningfulness that is so important to helpers in order to continue doing a good job.

Home helpers and recipients seem to have the same conception of what care entails. Asked about their understanding of the conception, most respondents, home helpers, and recipients alike said that care consists of both a *physical help aspect* (*tedasuke*/help with practical tasks that the recipient no longer manages alone) and *a psychological aspect* or the human relationship. One Japanese helper put it this way: 'Care is not only about the physical aspect, but also about feelings...To help them see how they can live every single day, so that they can think that every day is worth living.' In other words, *kaigo*/care also means to care about and to be sensitive towards the recipients' state of being and needs, so that they can feel secure and comfortable. This is at the crux of what relational power is in practice. Looking at home helpers' work in this way makes us realize just how important their work is, and that structural power should be employed to secure sufficient space for relational power.

Appendix

See Table 5.5.

Table 5.5: Content of work (%)

How often do home helpers...	Japan	Norway
Clean recipient's home		
Daily	41	74
Weekly	53	17
More seldom	3	10
Never	3	
Make lunch or dinner for recipient		
Daily	27	25
Weekly	53	11
More seldom	6	12
Never	14	52
Go shopping for recipient		
Daily	19	6
Weekly	60	30
More seldom	12	27
Never	9	38
Help with bathing		
Daily	8	16
Weekly	47	26
More seldom	10	6
Never	35	52
Wash clothes for recipient		
Daily	15	15
Weekly	53	44
More seldom	13	33
Never	19	8
Accompany to medical doctor		
Daily	3	1
Weekly	19	4
More seldom	44	32
Never	34	64
Accompany for a walk or to shop		
Daily	4	0
Weekly	32	3
More seldom	25	23
Never	39	74
Have a cup of coffee/tea with the recipient		
Daily	1	3
Weekly	14	16
More seldom	16	59
Never	68	23
Make bed/clean sheets for recipient		
Daily	11	50
Weekly	58	40
More seldom	21	10
Never	10	0

Chapter 6
Care Providers in Japan: The Potential of and Challenges for Social Enterprises

Yayoi Saito

(Translated by Beverley Anne Yamamoto)

Introduction

I discussed some characteristics of home help development in Japan in Chapter 3. When we look at the history of elderly care in Japan, we see that the Japanese care system was strongly centralized and bureaucratic. In this chapter I discuss some potentials of user and worker participation in care services.

Since the 1980s the theories of new public management and welfare mix have had widespread influence throughout Europe in the field of welfare. A cross-national comparison shows that since the 1990s there has been a growing trend towards the introduction of both private consignment for care services and voucher systems. This is true even in the Scandinavian countries that had hitherto been noted for providing welfare services through the public sector. For example, in large cities in Sweden there are already municipalities where more than 50% of care services are provided by private enterprises. This wave of quasi-marketization of care services has also exerted a strong influence on the Japanese elderly care system.

In Japan the Long-term Care Insurance (LTCI) System (*Kaigo hoken seido*) was introduced in April 2000. Users are not only able to choose the type of service, but also the service provider. Before the introduction of the LTCI System, almost all care services were provided either by corporations licensed by the Ministry of Health and Welfare, and Labour—so-called social welfare corporations (*Shakai fukushi hōjin*) (see section below)—or directly by local municipalities. From a legal point of view, social welfare corporations are private bodies, but they are highly dependent on public resources to operate. As a result, there is ambiguity over whether the services they provide constitute public or private sector services.

In the 1990s senior citizens' homes managed by private enterprises (for-profit corporations) began to be established. Receiving no public assistance, these facilities were based on a contractual relationship between the service provider in the market and the users. When compared to this type of care service set up entirely within a market contract system, those offered by social welfare corporations appear to be of a primarily public nature.

When social welfare corporations construct new facilities for the elderly, they receive subsidies from the central government and the local municipality to cover approximately two-thirds of the costs. Operating expenses are likewise covered by measures taken by the state and local municipalities. In addition, the tax system clearly treats social welfare corporations favorably.

Social enterprises in the care sector, one of the subjects of this chapter, have been greatly influenced by the NPO Law (*Tokutei hieiri katsudō sokushin hō*) (see below) that came into effect in 1998. In Japan informal, voluntary activities were already being carried out on a regional level before this. Such voluntary services included assisting elderly persons living alone with domestic chores and a meals-on-wheels-type lunch delivery service.

The NPO Law paved the way for such informal activities to be socially re-evaluated as formal activities. For example, a voluntary group that had been organizing recreational activities for elderly people with dementia several times a week in their homes could, as a result of the NPO Law, now become a formal service provider by acquiring corporate body status. As a result of this new status, it became possible for these groups to be commissioned to carry our projects by the local municipality and become LTCI providers, and so the number of groups with stable finances for their activities increased.

Against this social background, the aims of this chapter are fourfold: first, to highlight the structural characteristics of care service providers from a historical point of view before the LTCI System was introduced. Second, to show how the structural situation of, and conditions faced by, care service providers has been changed by the LTCI System. In particular, this chapter analyzes the changed conditions surrounding provision of long-term care by providers generally and demonstrates variations between prefectures. It also shows the types of corporations active in the care service market. Third, based on my own fieldwork, to analyze the potential of NPO care providers as social enterprises. Finally, to elucidate the importance of NPO providers in the care sector in Japan, as well as to point to some of the challenges they face.

Care providers before the LTCI System

Table 6.1 shows the difference between the current LTCI System and the former system. Before the LTCI System was introduced in 2000, the system

Table 6.1: Differences between new and former systems in elderly care (Japan)

	Former system (to March 31, 2000)		New system (from April 1, 2000)
	Social Welfare System for the Elderly (*Rōjin fukushi seido*)	**Health Insurance System for the Elderly (*Rōjin hoken seido*)**	**Long-Term Care Insurance System (*Kaigo hoken seido*)**
Year	April 1963	April 1983	April 2000
Main laws	Law for the Welfare of the Elderly (*Rōjin fukushi hō*)	Health and Medical Services Law for the Elderly (*Rōjin hoken hō*)	Long-term Care Insurance Law (*Kaigo hoken hō*)
Funding system	Tax	Insurance	Insurance
Service target	Elderly with low-incomes, living alone or with other special requirements	Those aged seventy years old and over and those between sixty-five and seventy with disabilities	All elderly
Eligibility for service	Care needs and conditions of family structure, income, etc.	Care needs	Care needs
Co-payment from user	According to ability to pay	530 yen/visit, 1,200 yen/day of hospitalization	10% of service fee
Care service providers	Social welfare corporations and local governments	Medical corporations (mainly)	Public and private providers
Services	In-home services (home help, day care services, etc.). Facilities (Special Nursing Home for the Elderly, etc.).	In-home services (home-visiting nurse). Facilities (Health Service Facilities for the Elderly).	In-home services. Services at facilities.
User choice	No	Yes	Yes

Source: Nishimura (1998) and supplemented by author.

for elderly care in Japan was divided into two areas. One was the Social Welfare System for the Elderly (*Rōjin fukushi seido*) and the other was the Health Insurance System for the Elderly (*Rōjin hoken seido*). The Social Welfare System for the Elderly was regulated by the Law for the Welfare of the Elderly (*Rōjin fukushi hō*), which was enacted in 1963. As the number of elderly began to increase, and some reform of the health insurance system was necessary, in 1983 the government passed the Health and Medical Services Law for the Elderly (*Rōjin hoken hō*), which regulated the Health Insurance

System for the Elderly. To a certain extent, this represented a reform of the health insurance system.

The Social Welfare System for the Elderly was run on the basis of tax payments, and fitted into a framework of *poor relief.* For example, public services in this system were aimed at elderly people with low incomes and no family support (see Chapter 3). It was difficult to gain a place in Special Nursing Homes (*Tokubetsu yōgo rōjin hōmu*) for elderly with family support and/or income from a pension because of the limited number of Special Nursing Homes (facilities that by law provide nursing care to bedridden people over sixty-five years of age). Most residents in Special Nursing Homes were from low-income groups and were not required to pay fees. Service providers in this system were limited to social welfare corporations and local governments, and service users or their families had no choice within this system.

The Health Insurance System for the Elderly was run on the basis of insurance premiums and contributions. This system was quite different from the social welfare system; service fees were the same for all users, and users could choose services and service providers. Service providers were mainly medical corporations (*Iryō hōjin*).

In this section I have outlined some of the primary characteristics of the former system and care service providers. With this background knowledge, we can now move on to see how much the Japanese elderly care system has changed as a result of the introduction of the LTCI System.

Social welfare corporations (*Shakai fukushi hōjin*)

Care providers in Japan were characterized by the Social Welfare Services Law (*Shakai fukushi jigyō hō*), which was revised and the name changed to the Social Welfare Law (*Shakai fukushi hō*) in 2000. The Social Welfare Service Law was a comprehensive welfare administration law enacted in 1951 that defined the scope and nature of all major public and private welfare agencies (Nakamura 1981: 13).

The law permitted only government and social welfare corporations to work as welfare service providers. The Social Welfare Services Law gave special status to social welfare corporations as welfare service providers. According to Article 22 of the law, social welfare corporations were private welfare administrative organizations and they could be accredited to provide specified publicly recognized welfare services and to receive public financing for these programs.

Why were social welfare corporations established? One reason is that the Japanese Constitution (*Nippon-koku Kempō*), enacted in 1945, prohibited religious or charitable organizations from receiving public funds. Article 89 of the Constitution states that 'no public money or other property shall be expended or appropriated for the use, benefit, or maintenance of any religious institution or association, or for any benefit or maintenance of any religious institution or association, or for any charitable, educational, or benevolent enterprises not under the control of public authority.'

After the Second World War, many groups, including churches, temples, and voluntary organizations, tried to provide welfare services in Japan, but if they wanted to start residential services with public funding, it was necessary to be accredited as a social welfare corporation. Public funds (*sochi-hi*) were provided on the basis of a standard per capita allowance per month per person, paid to institutions in which users were placed under the authority of welfare legislation (Nakamura 1981: 20). These funds were usually allocated at the ratio of 80% from the national government, with the remaining 20% variously divided between prefecture and municipality, depending on the type of care involved (Nakamura 1981: 20).

Social welfare corporations were private organizations according to the law, but they were strictly controlled by the government. Many voluntary organizations that were active in the early post-war period were accredited as social welfare corporations. While they benefited from having a stable source of income for their organizational management, some organizations lost the spirit of charity and voluntarism that was their initial strength (Tsutsui 2003: 20).

Social welfare councils *(Shakai fukushi kyōgi kai*) have played quite an important role as care service providers in Japan, especially in some rural area, and are accredited as social welfare corporations. The National Council of Social Welfare (*Zenkoku shakai fukushi kyōgi kai*) was incorporated as a social welfare corporation in 1951. Its purpose was to promote and organize the activities of voluntary social work organizations throughout the country. In the 1960s and 1970s, all of the forty-seven prefectures and most of the municipalities had organized social welfare councils. They emerged as one kind of social welfare corporation, and were important providers of care services from the 1980s, especially in rural areas. Even now we can find some areas where a social welfare council is the only care service provider.

The Social Welfare System for the Elderly (*Rōjin fukushi seido*)

A number of important laws relating to welfare were enacted in the early post-war period. Six fundamental laws concerning social welfare were passed around this time, and are referred to as the six basic welfare laws (*fukushi roppō*). The Social Welfare Services Law (1951), mentioned above, provides the basis for present-day welfare service delivery in Japan. In addition, the six basic welfare laws are the Daily Life Security Law (*Seikatsu hogo hō*) (enacted 1946, revised 1950), the Child Welfare Law (*Jidō fukushi hō*) (1947), the Law for the Welfare of Physically Disabled Persons (*Shintaishōgaisha fukushi hō*) (1949), the Law Concerning Mental Health and Welfare for Mentally Disabled (*Seishinhakujyakusha fukushi hō*) (1950, amended 1993), the Law for the Welfare of the Elderly (1963), and the Law for Maternal and Child Welfare (*Boshi fukushi hō*) (1964).

The Law for the Welfare of the Elderly is one of the six basic welfare laws. This law provides such services for the elderly as physical support for the so-called 'golden age clubs' (*rōjin kai*), and all services that are not provided for under more general legislation. Residential services also are regulated by the Law for the Welfare of the Elderly. For example, Special Nursing Homes for the Elderly and Homes for the Elderly (*yōgo rōjin hōmu*, which provide care for people over sixty-five who have limited financial resources but are basically in good health but unable to live in their own homes) are defined and provided for by this law. Only social welfare corporations can be providers for these services.

The Health Insurance System for the Elderly (*Rōjin hoken seido*)

There is a consensus that health care insurance achieved a universal level in 1961 in Japan. In other words, the coverage of the medical insurance system expanded to all Japanese people through the new National Health Insurance Law (*Shin-Kokumin hoken hō*).

National Health Insurance (*Kokumin kenkō hoken*) is a government-sponsored contributory health insurance program, primarily for those not covered by employee-type health insurance. Insured members include self-employed business owners, farmers, part-time workers, students, and retired people. Nevertheless, by the 1980s the National Health Insurance System was facing serious financial difficulties, in part because retired people had come to occupy such a large percentage of all the insured members. To introduce fairer cost sharing of medical care by the elderly, the Health and Medical Services Law for the Elderly was enacted in 1983.

The Health and Medical Services Law for the Elderly was revised in 1986 to introduce institutional health care services for the elderly. This kind of institutional care was called the Health Service Facility for the Elderly (*Rōjin hoken shisetsu*). It provided residential services that included both medical care and daily living services in an attempt to facilitate a patient's return to a normal life at home. These services were intended for the elderly and other people whose health was in the recovery stage or stabilization period and who needed medical care with an emphasis on rehabilitation and nursing/personal care, rather than inpatient medical treatment. It was expected that the facilities would play a role as intermediate entities between homes and hospitals. The Health and Medical Services Law for the Elderly was revised again in 1991, and home-visit nursing care services were introduced.

Medical corporations have been the main service providers of both Health Service Facilities for the Elderly and home-visit nursing. Medical corporations can be formed for the purpose of establishing hospitals, clinics, or health care facilities for the elderly, and are regulated by the Medical Services Law (*Iryō hō*).

Pluralism among service providers and social enterprises

Service expansion and user choice

Table 6.2 shows the number of long-term care service users. The number of users, especially of in-home services, increased rapidly over a six–year period. In April 2000, when the LTCI System was introduced, 970,000 elderly people used in-home services. Six years later this figure had risen to 2,510,000. Such dramatic expansion was unexpected. Pluralism among service providers has worked to bring about this situation.

Under the LTCI System users can choose care services and providers. A care needs assessment (see Table 3.5) is necessary for all elderly who want to make use of care services. The elderly are categorized into eight groups (including 'independent') on the basis of this assessment. Each group has its own monthly upper limit on costs, and users can choose services within this assigned budget.

Table 6.3 shows services in the system. As a mechanism to support the decisions of users, there are specialists (care managers) who can formulate service plans (care plans) and coordinate the selected services with the service providers. For services in the category of in-home services, users can enjoy some choice. But in the category of services at facilities, care service providers are limited.

New providers of in-home services

Article 2 of the LTCI Law specifies that care services should be provided by a diverse range of service providers and institutions, and that it is expected that a large number of private businesses will enter the market.

A contractual way of thinking was introduced into the LTCI System. Through to this point, the government had made decisions unilaterally concerning administrative measures regarding people in need of care. Now,

Table 6.2: The number of long-term care service users (1000 people)

	April 2000	April 2001	April 2002	June 2005
In-home services	970	1,420	1,720	2,510
Facility services	520	650	690	780
Total	1,490	2,070	2,410	3,290

Source: Ministry of Health, Labour, and Welfare 2007.

Table 6.3: Care services offered within the LTCI System

In-home services	*Services at facilities*
Home-visit care (home helper services) Home-visit nurse (home nursing) Day long-term care (day services) Short stay long-term care (short stay services) Community life care for persons with dementia (group living for the elderly with dementia)	Long-term care at welfare facilities for the elderly (Special Nursing Homes for the Elderly) Long-term care at health facilities for the elderly (Health Service Facilities for the Elderly) Long-term care at medical care facilities at a sanatorium
Pluralism among service providers	Social welfare corporations, medical corporations

however, the user makes a contract with the service provider, and this has become the centerpiece of the LTCI System. The role of the government is not to produce services, but to specialize in managing the LTCI System through certification of long-term care need (local municipalities), designation of service providers (prefectural-level government), and by managing the public finances of the LTCI System for the insurers (local municipality). It is a kind of *purchaser–provider model* (see Chapter 3).

With implementation of the LTCI System, new providers such as for-profit corporations (*Eiri hōjin*), NPO corporations (NPO *hōjin*) (see below), agricultural cooperatives (*Nōgyō Kyōdō Kumiai*), and cooperative associations (*Seikatsu Kyōdō Kumiai*) have set up new care service businesses.

Table 6.4 shows the variation that exists in terms of care providers and the increase in their numbers. The number of care providers has been increasing, especially in-home services. The growth in for-profit corporations and NPO corporations is outstanding.

A comparison of the period immediately following the introduction of the LTCI System (April 2000) with a period five years later (May 2005) reveals

Table 6.4: Changes in in-home care service providers (2001 and 2005)

Category of provider	May 2001	May 2005	Rate of increase
Social welfare corporations			
Other than social welfare councils	15 ,134	19,838	31%
Social welfare councils	4,884	5,132	5%
Medical corporations	42,907	61,093	42%
Public interest corporations	2,666	3,310	24%
For-profit corporations	21,882	50,585	131%
NPO corporations	682	27 35	301%
Agricultural cooperatives	952	1,189	25%
Cooperative associations	1,401	1,966	40%
Local governments	5,384	6,416	19%
Total	95,892	152 264	59%

Source: Ministry of Health, Labour, and Welfare 2007.

the following three characteristics. First, there has been a rapid increase in the number of for-profit corporations among providers. The rate of increase was 131% during this period. Second, NPO corporations, categorized here as social enterprises, increased almost three times. Furthermore, the number of NPO corporations involved in providing day care services and managing group homes for senior citizens suffering from dementia also increased. Third, there has been a decline in the hitherto core role played by social welfare corporations and service providers directly managed by municipal bodies.

Under the former system these groups carried out care services completely from their own sources of funding. As a result, there was a heavy financial burden for users of home-help services and private nursing homes provided by for-profit corporations, and usage of such services was restricted to those who had the ability to shoulder these expenses themselves. Users were also at high risk of a company becoming bankrupt.

Services offered by organizations such as NPO corporations, agricultural cooperatives, and cooperative associations were supported by the labor of unpaid or lowly remunerated volunteers, and, being small in scale, there were limits to how much services could expand and to the number of elderly they could cater to.

Since the introduction of the LTCI System, all providers receive remuneration for care services offered on the basis of the same standard. Private nursing homes run by for-profit corporations have become an option for middle-income groups because of the lower financial burden that users now

Table 6.5: In-home care providers (December 2000, Shiga Prefecture)

Type of care service provider	Number of providers	Share of services (%)
Municipalities	18 (4.1%)	10.9
Social welfare corporations	210 (47.9%)	56.5
Medical corporations	38 (8.6%)	14.2
For-profit corporations	135 (30.9%)	10.9
NPO corporations	8 (1.8%)	1.0
Agricultural cooperatives	9 (2.0%)	0.5
Cooperative associations	2 (0.4%)	0.1
Others	18 (4.1%)	6.0
Total	438 (100%)	100%

Source: Saito 2001.

have to shoulder. Management of such private nursing homes has become more stable, and the risk of bankruptcy has been reduced. It is now possible for NPO corporations to operate from a stable financial base as remuneration for care provision has become a new source of finance.

When looking at the number of care service providers, we have to pay attention to service share. Table 6.5 shows an example of Shiga Prefecture (1.39 million people). Looking at the number of care service providers that are for-profit organizations, we can see that they account for 30.9% of all providers. At the same time, if we look at the share of services, we find that for-profit organizations provide only 10.9% of total services. This means that the number of providers does not translate directly into service share. Thus more traditional providers, such as social welfare corporations, still play an important role as service providers in some areas.

Regional differences in the extent of the pluralization of service providers

To what extent is there variation by region in the pluralization of service providers? Figure 6.1 shows the diversification in the number of designated home-help care providers by major corporate body type. As can be seen, the degree of diversification in home-help care service providers varies greatly across the forty-seven prefectures and metropolitan administrative districts in Japan (Saito 2005: 313–15).

Overall we can divide the forty-seven prefectures and metropolitan administrative regions in Japan into two main clusters. First, there are municipalities where the majority of service providers are for-profit corporations. Second, there are municipalities that rely overwhelmingly on

Figure 6-1: Pluralization of care providers (home help services) in some example areas (············ 2000 and ——— 2004)

Commercial companies are active in some big cities

Tokyo

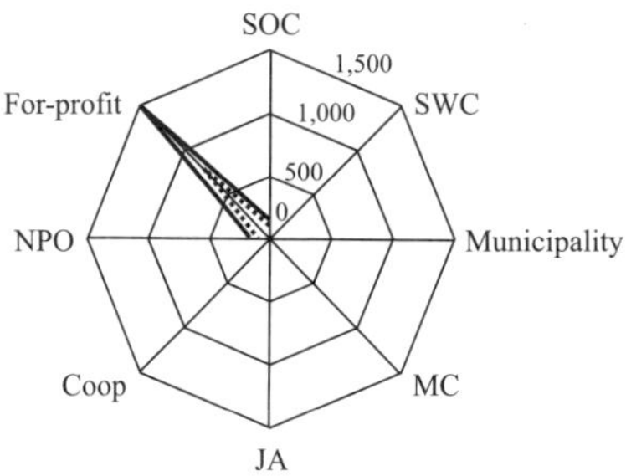

Chiba

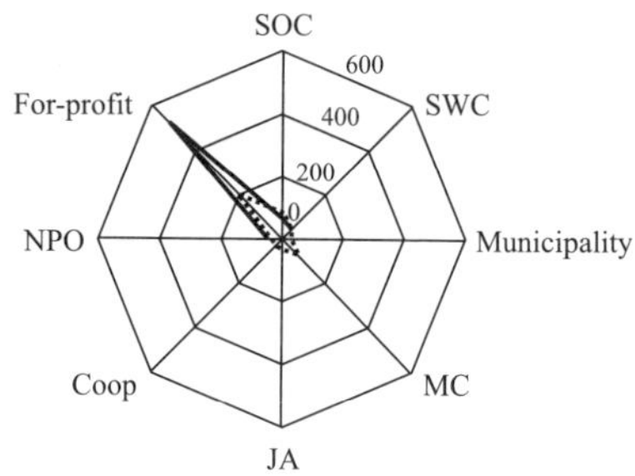

Social welfare corporations still have a large role in some rural areas

Kagoshima

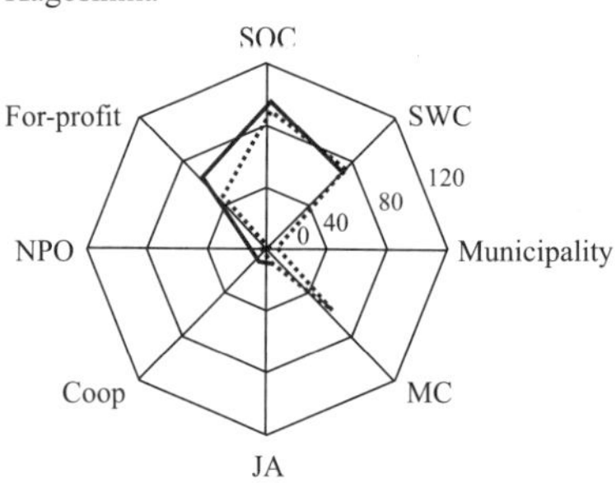

Shimane

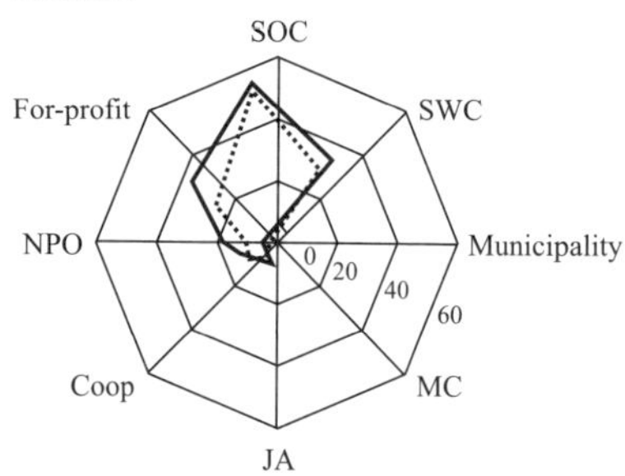

Social welfare councils are active in some specially designated rural areas

Nagano

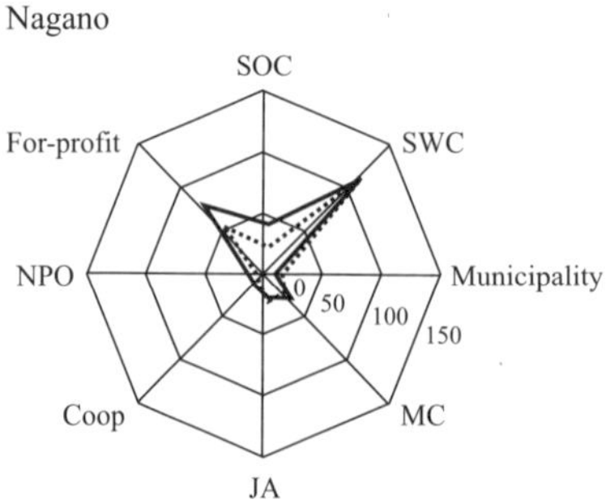

Tottori

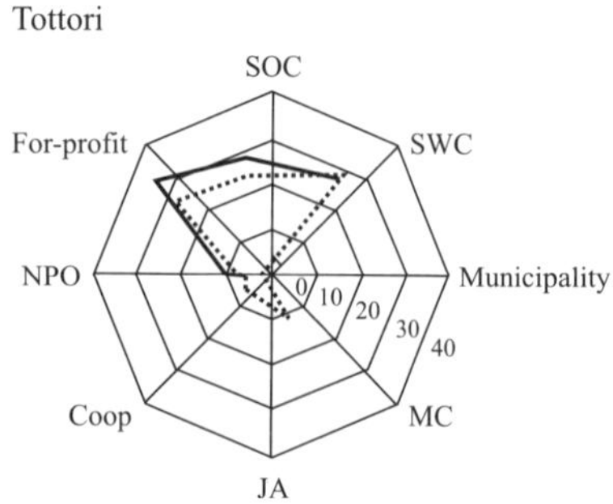

Figure 6-1: Continued

SOC: Social welfare corporations (*Shakai fukushi hōjin*)
SWC: Social welfare councils (*Shakai fukushi kyōgi kai)*
Municipality: Self-governing municipal bodies
MC: Medical corporations (*Iryō hōjin*)
JA: Agricultural cooperatives (*Nogyō Kyōdō kumiai*)
Coop: Cooperative associations (*Seikatsu Kyōdō kumiai*)
NPO: NPO corporations (*NPO hōjin*)
For-profit: For-profit corporations (*Eiri hōjin*)

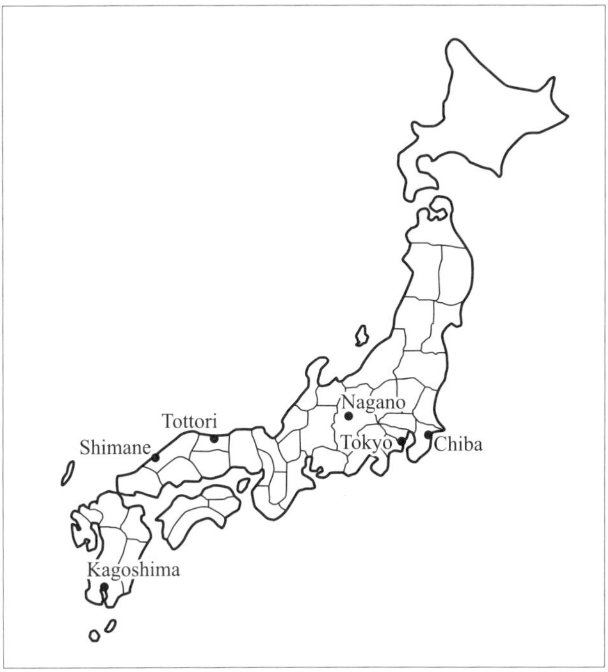

the social welfare corporation model for the delivery of such services (Saito 2005: 316).

Tokyo Metropolitan Area and Chiba Prefecture, followed by Kanagawa, Saitama, and Hyogo and Osaka prefectures have many municipalities where the majority of home-help care services are provided by for-profit corporations. The main characteristic of such prefectures and administrative areas is that they are largely urban. Indeed, they include prefectures with some of the largest Japanese cities (Saito 2005: 316).

Municipalities with a large number of services provided by social welfare corporations include those in relatively rural Shimane, Aomori, Saga, and Miyazaki prefectures. In these regions the overall number of service providers has increased, but social welfare corporations have remained the main service suppliers. Municipalities with large numbers of services provided by social welfare corporations are those with a large number of depopulated areas such as Shimane and Aomori prefectures, and the prefectures in Kyushu (Saito 2005: 316).

In terms of social welfare corporations, there are also municipalities where social welfare councils play a substantive role. In Nagano and Tottori prefectures there are municipalities with an extremely high number of social welfare councils. Municipalities where there are more social welfare councils than other social welfare corporations are in Akita, Fukui, Niigata, Fukushima, Yamanashi, Gifu, Hokkaido, Shiga, and Ehime prefectures.

In addition to this, municipalities that are notable for the participation of medical corporations are areas with a large number of hospitals, such as Kochi, Oita, Kumamoto, Tokushima, and Okinawa prefectures. Not surprisingly, municipalities where agricultural cooperatives play a significant role in care provision are the agricultural prefectures such as Iwate, Ishikawa, and Toyama (Saito 2005: 316).

Japanese social enterprises in elderly care—a fact-finding survey

This section considers the situation of NPO corporations as new care service providers in the LTCI System based on my fieldwork.

Social enterprises and their contributions

In European counntries there is an interest in the potential of the social economy and an appreciation of the contribution of social enterprises in the provision of social services appears.

According to Pestoff, social enterprises are bodies that try to fulfill several goals simultaneously, recognizing that no single goal can constantly be maximized, but rather that several of them can be satisfactorily fulfilled at the same time. Social enterprises do not exist to maximize the return on capital nor revenue over expenses; rather, they are willing to accept a lower, but nevertheless satisfactory, economic return on their efforts. They do this in order to combine the necessary economic goal with other important social goals that can also be achieved or satisfied (Pestoff 1998: 13).

Pestoff indicates three potential contributions that can be made by social enterprises. First, workers are highly motivated and their working lives are enriched (Pestoff 1998: 15). The model of the worker cooperative, in particular, has an empowering effect on workers. This model offers workers many opportunities to be involved in decision making and increases the possibility that they will be able to make decisions within the workplace. In turn, the high satisfaction level of the staff translates into an improvement in the quality of the services (Pestoff 1998: 187).

Second, social enterprises contribute towards the empowerment of service users (Pestoff 1998: 15). This is particularly the case with users' cooperatives where responsibility is accepted for the service produced due to the fact that it is the result of the cooperative effort of the users themselves. Within this framework, if the user wants to see an improvement in the quality of the service, all he or she needs to do is verbalize his or her dissatisfaction and ask for the matter to be addressed (Pestoff 1998: 208–09).

Third, social enterprises also contribute to a variety of social value (Pestoff 1998: 15). There is flexibility of service provision. The expectation of social enterprises is that they will not only provide social care services for the elderly, their primary objective, but will also potentially contribute, as a secondary objective, to the creation of social value in a variety of ways (Pestoff 1998: 104–05).

NPO corporations in Japan as social care enterprises

The Law to Promote Specified Non-profit Activities (the NPO Law, 1998) provides corporate status to voluntary organizations. According to the NPO Law, an NPO should contribute to the advancement of the interests of many people and their activities. Twelve areas are stressed: health, medical care, and welfare; social education; community development; culture; the arts and sports; the environment; disaster relief; community safety; human rights and peace; international cooperation; equal treatment of women in society; sound nurturing of youth; and support of any of the above.

As of 2009, 37,785 organizations are certificated by the NPO Law, and 57.7% of these work as service providers in health, medical care, and welfare (Cabinet Office, Government of Japan 2009).

Is it possible to regard NPO service providers as social enterprises? To answer this question, I carried out a survey of NPO corporations in elderly care in 2004.

Table 6.6 shows the requirements considered necessary to regard an organization as a social enterprise by some researchers (Kobe Research Institute of Urban Issues 2002: 35). A social enterprise needs to meet five requirements regarding its business standing, community-based character, creativity, citizenship, and regional contributions. Before the LTCI System

Table 6.6: Requirements for community-based social enterprises

Components	Requirements
Business standing	Have an independent business income in the form of a guaranteed major source of continuous income.
Community	Carry out business activities in a specific target area.
Creativity	As part of business content and objectives, engage in activities that seek solutions to local community problems.
Citizenship	Guarantee the agency of the local citizens sector, including local citizens, in terms of financing and operations when new businesses are developed by them.
Regional contribution	Contribute unambiguously to the solution of local problems.

Source: Kobe Research Institute of Urban Issues 2002: 35.

was introduced, there were a lot of voluntary groups working in elderly care. While they contributed to society, they did not meet the above requirements. A lack of stable funding makes it impossible for them to offer continuous, stable services. The NPO Law and the LTCI System has provided these groups with the opportunity to become independent service providers with some kind of social value.

Case studies of NPO corporations as social enterprises

For my field research into social care enterprises in 2004 (Saito 2005), 'A' Prefecture in the western part of Japan was chosen as a research field. The primary reason for choosing this prefecture was the variation seen within it. There is an area being developed as a dormitory town, an industrial area with large factories, a mountainous region designated by the government as a heavy snowfall area, and a prosperous agricultural area. Given that the region combines such diversity, we should be able to see clearly how local characteristics impact upon the activities of social care enterprises. The second reason for choosing this prefecture was that the number of NPO corporations was higher than in other prefectures. It means NPO corporations are active in the area.

Organizations deemed to be social enterprises were chosen from service providers that had been covered in daily and local newspaper stories shortly after the introduction of the LTCI System in April 2000. Organizations were chosen as target enterprises on the basis that they (1) worked in different areas, (2) represented different corporate body statuses, and (3) provided different services. In total twelve providers were selected; of these, three providers declined to participate in the study on the basis that they were too busy. Finally, nine organizations supported my field research.

Here I pick up two cases among these nine research samples.

A case of NPO corporation 'A'

NPO 'A' was established in 1991. It was accredited as an NPO corporation in 2002, and became a care service provider of the LTCI System. It provides home help services and day care services, which are targeted at Korean residents. The organization has a strong mission to help elderly from Korea.

Business aspect

When it started its work at the beginning of the 1990s, NPO 'A' had little money for its activities. The municipality provided some subsidy, but staff members were not sufficiently paid. After becoming a care provider of the LTCI, the NPO was able to employ paid staff, and it had its own office. The approximate annual turnover is 12 million yen (EUR90,500/US$133,300). It is a small business, but the money from the insurance helps to provide stable management.

Community

NPO 'A' works in and for a Korean community in the municipality.

Creativity

Some Korean elderly who stay in Japan do not speak Japanese. Communication difficulties sometimes hinder Korean elderly from joining mainstream day care services. Care workers who work in NPO 'A' speak both Japanese and Korean. They also cook Korean food for the elderly. Users are satisfied with such services, and become healthier. Workers also enjoy working for them.

Citizenship

Almost all staff and volunteers live in the same municipality as the users.

Regional contribution

NPO 'A' is not only a care provider, but also works towards intercultural communication in the community. It tries to have some meetings and activities, and to contribute useful information and news concerning daily life to Korean residents.

A case of NPO corporation 'B'

NPO 'B' works in a rural area, from where members of the younger generation leave to go to the big cities. Some middle-aged residents established NPO

'B' to cheer up their town. They tried to make a small business of elderly care because they have a lot of elderly in their area.

NPO 'B' was accredited as a NPO corporation in 2002, and became a care service provider of the LTCI in 2003. It provides home help services and day care services in the LTCI System. Besides these services, it provides some small welfare services, which are contracted out by the municipality.

NPO 'B' has a strong mission to activate and empower the old town.

Business aspect

NPO 'B' has an approximate annual turnover of 10 million yen (EUR75,400/ US$111,000). It is a small business, and has an office for its activities.

Community

NPO 'B' works in a small community in a rural area.

Creativity

It aims to revitalize the town in cooperation with members of the local Chamber of Commerce and Industry (*Syōkō kaigisyo*). It has succeeded in creating small businesses such as its 'Shopping Service for Elderly.' In this service, shop clerks deliver goods to frail elderly, who shop via the telephone.

Citizenship

Almost all staff and volunteers live in the same area as users.

Regional contribution

The NPO undertakes unprofitable businesses such as shopping services. It also provides after-school care of disabled children. As these are quite small tasks with small subsidies from the municipality, no one else wanted to provide such services. NPO 'B' also contributes to job creation.

Analysis of research results—social value

The results and an analysis of this research appears in an earlier paper (Saito 2005). In the following section I provide an outline of this. I verify that social enterprises produce social value over and above that related to care services, and highlight the challenges faced by social care enterprises working in the care sector in Japan.

Playing a role in sustainable community revitalization

The goal of social enterprises working in the care sector is not simply to provide care services. There are cases where care businesses are initiated to allow the group to be involved in a sustained way with civic activities such as those addressing environmental problems, community revitalization, and community activities. With the LTCI System in the background, it is easy to set up a business as a care provider. Thus, we can see that some groups become care providers in order to secure the organization's financing for civic activities.

Implementation of small-scale services

There are examples of local municipalities commissioning social enterprises to provide care services on a very small scale (perhaps only one or two people) where it would be difficult due to the small numbers involved for them to provide the care services themselves. One example is after-school care of disabled children. This scenario is particularly likely in depopulated areas.

Discovery of new challenges

Social care enterprises can respond to the needs of elderly people with special needs. For example, there has been little debate to date in Japan concerning the need for care services targeting foreign residents. Social care enterprises have discovered a variety of new challenges for the care sector such as elderly foreign residents suffering from dementia who have difficulties communicating in Japanese, and the difficulties faced by foreign residents when it comes to using existing day care services, which are aimed primarily at Japanese people.

The democracy and transparency of organizations

If we look at the structure and management of the board of directors of social enterprises in the care sector, we find they are composed of people who were involved in community activities before starting up businesses as care providers, and many are local residents. Due to the fact that they live locally and the small scale of the organizations, it is easy for board members to meet and board meetings are lively affairs. In some cases staff meetings include staff members with disabilities, and a space is created for an exchange of opinions. When it comes to appointing new staff members, efforts are made to include the views of all staff.

Table 6.7 summarizes the results of an interview survey concerning the potential contribution of social enterprises in the care sector.

It can be seen from the survey on social enterprises operating in the care sector that the democratic basis and transparency of the organizations are

Table 6.7: Social contribution of social enterprises – survey results

Social contribution (by Pestoff)	Results of the research
Work motivation and satisfaction of staff	Low staff turnover rate and low absentee rates
User empowerment	High user satisfaction level Increased user vitality/health Exchange and cooperation with the local community and local residents
Reaction of and contribution to social value	Dealing with special needs (e.g. depopulated areas, foreign residents) Regional spillover effect (e.g. job creation, local development) Creation of pioneering models

major factors in the high motivation of the staff. In all the organizations visited, staff members were working with enthusiasm.

Pestoff notes that due to the social-political processes inherent in these organizations, social enterprises expand possibilities for self-determination and control of one's work, as well as encourage the participation of staff in decision making. As a result, there exists the latent potential for a stressful job to be transformed into active work (Pestoff 1998: 239). This was true of the organizations participating in this research study.

On this occasion I did not carry out interviews with users, but it would appear that democracy and transparency in an organization reduce the distance between users and providers. Pestoff highlighted the case of a social enterprise running a nursery school in which parents were able to actively influence the conditions surrounding the business. A similar situation occurred among the organizations targeted in this study. For example, service providers considered contact with the families to be very important, and there were numerous opportunities created (Pestoff 1998: 214–16).

Furthermore, when considering the creation of social value, there were cases where, as a result of becoming long-term care providers, social enterprises were able to become involved in sustained ways with community revitalization activities; were able to implement small-scale welfare programs that are important but often overlooked, such as after-school care for children with disabilities; and were able to provide services for elderly foreign residents. As Pestoff has indicated, if social enterprises increase their presence in the field of personal social services, they will rejuvenate the public sector and make a unique contribution that will surely enrich the welfare state (Pestoff 1998: 20). A new set of circumstances that was not seen within the framework of the former system has emerged.

Challenges faced by social enterprises in elderly care

Low-paid labor and the sustainability problem

One challenge faced by the social care enterprises surveyed was concern about sustainability. Nearly all the businesses surveyed expressed concern about whether they would be able to continue with their missions or not, and whether there would be successors to take them over. Rather than being a discrete problem, this insecurity surrounding the sustainability of the business can be viewed as an inherent organizational characteristic of social enterprises in the care sector.

The low pay of staff was offered as another reason for the feeling of unease about the sustainability of the business by a number of respondents. The activities of Japanese social enterprises in the care sector are to a large part supported by the strong sense of mission and the perseverance of staff.

According to Pestoff, as a result of privatization, which demands that the community shoulders a larger share of the responsibility, the provision of social services has become something subordinate (losing its autonomy) and thrust on the female labor force with a concomitant erosion of professionalism. Women have been separated from the regular employment market, discarded, and made unpaid providers of care services within the home. This has been the path of the welfare service privatization in Central and Eastern Europe. It is in this context that Pestoff expresses apprehension about the privatization and communitization of welfare services, including elderly care (Pestoff 1998: 248).

In Japan, unless one is free from worries about how to make a living and has a very strong sense of mission, it is quite difficult to choose a social enterprise in the care sector as one's place of work. This reality is tied in with the sense of insecurity concerning successors to continue the business.

Referring to a statement made by Adalbert Evers, Pestoff (1998: 53) states that:

> Evers argues that merely conceiving of voluntary organizations or cooperatives as cheap service providers due to volunteers or a work obligations, etc., completely misses the point. Organizations found in the third sector are more than just service providers. They have a role in preserving and cultivating public virtues like participation, solidarity, etc.; they also promote economic, political

> and social change through pressure group activities; and their experiments often serve as innovators in service delivery, etc.

Pestoff warns about the risks of 'colonization' of the third sector, with it becoming a low budget 'dumping' ground used to shoulder ever more of the burden if there is excessive communitization of service provision (Pestoff 1998: 53).

Simply praising the potential contributions that can be made by social enterprises in the care sector carries with it great risk. We must make sure that the sense of duty of those involved in social enterprises in the care sector is not exploited to provide low-cost services. For this reason, the improvement of workplace conditions for those working in the care sector is a huge challenge currently facing Japan.

The takeover of small-scale providers and the trend towards a market oligopoly

It is difficult for social enterprises in the care sector to survive market competition. In June 2007 the joint-stock company COMSN, the biggest private care service provider, was forced to discontinue business as a result of a corruption scandal.

COMSN had been a pioneer social enterprise working in the care sector in Japan. At the time of its establishment in 1987, it was a small-scale provider of home help services, but despite this it was the first business in Japan to provide round-the-clock, at-home care services. It gained widespread attention throughout Japan. At that time, there were no providers offering evening and late-night home help services, although a few offered home help services over the weekend.

COMSN studied the home help system in the Scandinavian countries and implemented a similar system in Japan. Subsequently, the company has had a profound influence on the Japanese home help system. The founder and director of COMSN, Mr Enomoto, wanted to spread the philosophy of round-the-clock, at-home care throughout Japan and gave enthusiastic speeches (Yamanoi and Saito 1994: 47). However, just before the implementation of the LTCI System, COMSN was taken over by a large worker dispatch agency. Social enterprises usually have a strong mission of social contribution, but it is difficult to maintain the same mission all the time.

At the time when the scandal came to light in June 2007, COMSN had 24,000 employees and 65,000 users, and was in receipt of approximately 2% of total LTCI payments. While primarily offering nationwide home help services, at the same time it had 1100 business offices (dispatch bases), and managed 190 group homes for elderly people suffering from dementia and 535 private nursing homes.

The scandal involved irregularities concerning staffing, such as the running of business offices without a manager (even though this is required by law) and the absence of somebody in charge of service provision (it is obligatory to allocate one for every ten home helpers). In addition, improper and inflated claims for care remuneration were discovered. The cost of improper claims is believed to have been 430,530,000 yen (about EUR3.2 million/US$4.8 million) nationwide.

As a result of these fraudulent acts, COMSN is not permitted to apply for a new license or renew its existing one as a care service provider, making it practically impossible for it to continue in business. As a result, COMSN is seeking buyers for its businesses nationwide. It is quite difficult to carry out its original intention in a competitive market.

Reliable supply and the role of the government

It is clear that when the care market is left uncontrolled, an oligopoly occurs at the hands of large providers, as can be seen from the example of Sweden in the 1990s. In Sweden the private sector accounted for no more that 8% of care provision in 2002, but 70% share of this market was held by just a few large companies (Socialstyrelsen 2003).

A pluralization of care providers causes market competition among a variety of businesses, leading to the creation of better services and reasonable prices. However, when no policies are introduced to regulate the care service market, small-scale providers are taken over by larger ones and a situation of market oligopoly occurs. With the market now dominated by a few large companies, competition declines to a minimum. In order to maintain a moderate level of competition in the care market, it is necessary for the government to play a role. It is necessary to introduce policies that favor small-scale businesses with regard to, for example, bid tendering.

When thinking about the reliable provision of care services, we need to question whether this should be entrusted solely to new private-sector providers. Social enterprises in the care sector that have expanded their businesses are usually pioneers, and there is a greater likelihood that they will provide services that reflect the special needs of the users. However, they do not possess the service provision resources to cover entire regions, and neither do they aim to do so. Further, even large businesses have to balance their budgets and if an aspect of the business is not profitable they will quickly withdraw that service.

For example, in the case of the COMSN scandal, it has been impossible to find providers to take over COMSN home help services in depopulated areas. There are some depopulated regions in Japan that, after the start of the LTCI System, abolished care services directly operated by the government or by social welfare councils and became fully dependent on COMSN for the supply of care services. The reason for this is that, due to the financial situation of the municipalities, this reliance on COMSN meant a reduction in costs.

In order to ensure sustained care service supply, it is absolutely necessary to nurture existing providers with strong roots in the area, such as services provided by social welfare councils.

We should be looking to social enterprises in the care sector with an eye not only to the possibilities of guaranteeing continued delivery of care services, but also for their contribution in terms of improving quality of service by activating the market.

Conclusion and future research tasks

Social enterprises in the care sector not only fulfill the transient function of providing care services, but also engage in activities that contribute to the creation of social value. Pestoff suggests that social enterprises can make three potential contributions, namely the motivation and satisfaction of staff, the empowerment of users, and the creation of social value. These three potential contributions can be observed in Japanese social enterprises working in the care sector. In this sense, it is clear that there are great expectations of social enterprises as new providers of care services.

Yet, at the same time, from an interview survey of social enterprises working in the care sector, it is clear that there is concern over the sustainability of these new businesses. In particular, there is concern about the likely impact of staff working conditions. The majority of social enterprises working in the Japanese care sector rely heavily on the sense of mission of those working in the field. As Evers and Pestoff have both pointed out, if the communitization of services in the name of privatization goes too far, there is a risk that the participation of women in the regular labor market will be hindered and, in addition to them being sought as unpaid or low paid welfare-sector labor, there will be a loss of welfare expertise at the point of delivery. In order to fully realize the potential contribution of social enterprises and to avoid any exploitation of the sense of mission of those working in care in order to create a low budget welfare system, there should be a speedy improvement of working conditions.

As happened in the case of COMSN and the corruption scandal, there is always the possibility that, even in the case of an organization that started out as a social enterprise providing care services, the quality of the service could change radically if taken over by a large company.

The businesses developed by social care enterprises in the care sector are often pioneering in character and are more likely to provide services based on the special needs of their users. Nevertheless, they are not able to provide services on a scale that would cover entire regions, and neither do they aim to do so. Where there is a diversity of supply, there is a need to fully understand the special characteristics of each service provider.

There has been a remarkable increase in the participation of new main suppliers such as for-profit companies and NPO corporations in the care field. There are new demands for measures that will keep the competition between these new service providers on an equal footing and debate concerning the need for policy measures that favor social welfare corporations in the form of subsidies and tax measures. In this age of service pluralism, it is important to consider the way that social welfare corporations work if the issue of sustainable provision of services is to be adequately addressed.

In order to create a society where the elderly and people with disabilities can live within the community, we need to think how to improve the quality of services and guarantee the sustainability of services. Future research will address these issues.

Acknowledgements

This article was prepared a part of presentation for Japan Program 2007 'Eldercare in Japan and Norway: Organization and Quality' at the NTNU (Norwegian University of Science and Technology) in Trondheim, Norway. I would like to thank Dr Paul Midford (Associate Professor of Political Science and Sociology, NTNU) and Ms Unni Edvardsen to invite me the program. And I also thank Dr John Creighton Campbell (Professor of Political Science, The University of Michigan) to give me valuable comments to revise the paper.

Chapter 7
Challenges for the Future of Public Care— A Lesson from Norway

Kari Wærness

I have been engaged in sociological research on care since the 1970s. For many years my main research field was the public home care services in the Nordic countries. Much of the research was defined as applied or policy research and the goal was all the time to do research that would really matter in policies and practices. My research was based on my experiences as a politician in my home municipality. These experiences made me recognize that dominant scientific perspectives in the political planning discourse on public care services were defective and inadequate. They did not describe the problems in the everyday world of care in a way that could give new ideas on how to organize public care services to make them better both for clients and carers.

The problems facing the public home care services in the Nordic countries today are at least as great as they were more than thirty years ago. Research by those of us who used what is called a *bottom-up* or an *everyday life* perspective on these services seems to have had very little, if any, influence on the many reforms and on the ideological changes these services have gone through during more than three decades. Instead, *the care friendly ethos* guiding the Nordic welfare state has weakened during the past decade (Wrede et al. 2008). In this Chapter, I present a short historical overview of the changes that may contribute somewhat to the understanding of why a multifaceted *care crisis*, has become a problem, even in the Nordic care-friendly modern welfare states. At the same time, such crises are discussed in most other modern societies, and in many developing countries the care problems are even greater.

The 1950s and 1960s: homemaking as a new ideology

When public home care services for the elderly became an issue of rapidly increasing interest in Nordic social policy in the 1950s and 1960s, what we could call the *homemaking culture* became a dominant ideology behind the organization of these services. At this time there already existed a public home-based service for families in the Nordic countries. In this family care service, professional education and full-time positions for all employees was an ideal that, to some extent, was realized (Simonen 1990; Wærness 1995). The new public home care service for the elderly was not, however, made a part of this earlier established, and to some extent professionalized, home care service, and the dominant ideology behind it was quite different. In Norway and Sweden middle-aged housewives willing to take part-time work were explicitly called upon to go into this new service. Informal rather than formal competence was emphasized. The following statement by the leader of the Public Poverty Care Administration in Stockholm in 1953 is indicative of commonly held ideas of the necessary qualifications for workers in this service: home helpers were to have 'the ordinary competence of a housewife and a honest will to help one's fellow-beings' (Szebehely 1995: 58). Another key aspect was that home help should preferably be organized as part-time work. Male Norwegian parliamentarians expressed similar views in the 1960s, and even if some female members of the Parliament expressed different views, the Norwegian public home help service for the elderly became established on the basis of this same ideology (Nordhus, Isaksen, and Wærness 1987: 77). Also, in Finland, where the home care service for families with children was more professionalized than in the other Nordic countries, former housewives taking a short training course for household tasks were the preferred labor force in the new public service for the elderly. In contrast to the other Nordic countries, however, in Finland this service became organized as full-time work.

The homemaking ideology implied that each home helper gave versatile help to a few clients who she came to know personally. The individual client was allotted a certain amount of hours of home help, the content of which was not specified. There existed, however, some written rules about a few household services and tasks that were not to be provided. In practice, a client's immediate needs became decisive for which kinds of help were given. In order to give good care, the home helpers often had to provide services that, according to the written rules, were not to be given. They also often used more time than the clients were allotted or for which the home helpers were paid.

The welfare of the individual elderly person had, in the 1950s and 1960s, become a new and important explicit premise in the political discussions on how public care services for the elderly should be organized (Nordhus, Isaksen, and Wærness 1987: ch. 4). The public home care service was the enterprise that was supposed to realize this new premise. In addition, the question of how to organize the home care services to make the most efficient use of resources became an issue of steadily growing importance for the political authorities in all Nordic countries from the 1970s. Both the premise of economic efficiency and of individual welfare had resulted in very negative evaluations of public institutional care. Public home help and home nursing services were defined as an alternative to institutional care—an alternative that was evaluated as being both more cost-efficient and more humane for most elderly unable to care for themselves in everyday life. Good public care was defined as care as *homelike* as possible. The organizational changes of the public care services that were needed according to this new ideology were not based on any solid empirical analyses. No one had tried to fathom if it was economically and socially possible to organize public care services according to this ideal of good care, independent of how much help the individual elderly needed and their family situations. Another neglected question was the extent to which this ideal was possible to be realized in a situation where the public home helpers would have labor contracts in line with those available to other employees in a modern welfare state. For some years this public service was able to meet the increasing demand without major problems by continually recruiting new home helpers among the middle-aged housewives who were willing to work without regular labor contracts.

The 1970s and the 1980s: increasing bureaucratization, standardization, professionalization, and institutionalization

After some years it became evident that the goal of organizing a public home care service fulfilling traditional norms for good individual care came into conflict with the general norms and rules for modern working life. These included regulated working hours and tasks, and possibilities for specialization and professionalization and for moving up in a job hierarchy.

Empirical studies (Liljeström and Özgalda 1980; Wærness 1978) had shown that the first generation of home helpers, the middle-aged and elderly housewives, did not seem to want their work to change according to these dominating norms in working life. What they wanted was more time with each client and more regular contact with other home helpers. In their view the personal commitment to their clients and the autonomous judgments they made in their daily work were the most satisfying elements of the job. In general they wanted the public home help service to be organized in such a way that they could give versatile and personal help and care to individual clients and, at the same time, belong to a strong collective of equal home helpers. After a few years, however, the home help services began to change in a direction very different from what this first generation of frontline workers wanted. A generational crisis in the home help service emerged first in Sweden, when the elderly and middle-aged housewives were gradually replaced by a younger generation of women who had some special education for the job. The younger women found that the realities of the job did not fit the descriptions they had received through their education. The result was that they did not become a stable labor force. Great organizational problems arose when the traditional housewives gradually disappeared from the service and the home helpers' rights as normal employees had to be taken into consideration.

Reforms of public management and the organization of municipal health and care services began in the 1980s. A pioneering study by sociologist Ritva Gough (1987) documents the great problems of implementing the new public care policy in one of Sweden's most *innovative* municipalities. Many of the same problems have, over the years, been documented in many other studies. I therefore want to present some of the main findings of this study. These results tell us that to a great extent the problems we are struggling with today are not new. They have existed since the Nordic public home care services started to be organized as normal wage labor.

Gough (1987) shows that contrary to the intentions of the new ideology of public care, the new services introduced divisions of labor based on greater collectivization and specializations of functions, and increased the time needed for planning, administration, and coordination of activities. These tendencies, which were basic reasons for the severe criticism of the traditional institutional care services, could now be observed in the new community service program. This finding, which has since been confirmed in so many other studies of the public home care services, documents that many of the negative traits in institutional care should not be seen as a result of institutionalization per se, but as a result of a greater problem connected to managing and organizing effective care for the elderly with the greatest needs for help and care.

The statistics pointed to the number of elderly who received home help, and the total number of paid working hours of home helpers increased during the 1980s. Still, home helpers tended to experience a decrease in the amount of personal assistance they were able to give to individual elderly. This was to a large extent due to the changing nature of the care needs of the elderly. During these years, placements in institutions were delayed longer. Thus, there was a steady increase in clients who were in need of more care and help due to increasing age. In addition, new clients with complex problems ranging from alcohol abuse to other psychosocial concerns were included in the service. This would have presumed a professional competence and guidance for home helpers whose formal qualifications to cope with such problems were often lacking:

> Use of time, making priorities among clients, adjusting demands to available resources and *especially developing continuity in…social relations between home helpers and the elderly are factors that have contributed to a highly problematic organization which cannot be overlooked in future programs* (Gough 1987: 216, my italics).

Continuity in these social relations could be seen as a core value in a care service that should be *homelike*. This value is most easily realized when the elderly client's need for help and care is not too comprehensive (i.e. for those whose need for public care mainly consists of help with specific household tasks and regular shorter visits to satisfy needs for personal care, social contact, and security, and help with more irregular errands or small practical problems in everyday life). Homelike care becomes much more difficult to realize when clients become dependent on help for daily personal hygiene and eating. When a growing proportion of clients over time become dependent on more comprehensive care and the home helpers at the same time are supposed to become normal wage workers, this value of continuity became nearly impossible to realize.

The changes in public home care during the 1980s in the Swedish municipality in Gough's study (Gough 1987: 197–8), listed below, are much the same as those we find documented in studies from other communities in the Nordic countries in the 1980s and 1990s (see, for instance, Christensen 1997; Szebehely 1995). The changes are:

1. A home helper's personal knowledge of her clients is no longer a self-evident quality of the service. It becomes lost as individual home helpers have a larger number of clients and work more often outside their own local community, and because the distribution of work and the regulation of working hours make it impossible for the majority of home helpers to have their own clients.
2. Home helpers are exposed to the same kind of organizational and efficiency trials as the rest of the public administration services, and their division of labor is developed according to patterns similar to those found in large health care institutions. The work methods evolve in more professional directions, in spite of intentions to avoid this.

3. The occupational roles in the professional organization are made distinct, and different work tasks are decided for different personnel groups. This creates inequalities in salaries and employment conditions among the personnel groups.
4. One implicit consequence of this change is new divisions between personnel on the one hand and clients and their relatives on the other.

More studies that documented an increasing gap between ideals and realities in public home care argued for trying to find new ways of organizing these services. I, myself, argued that care work is based on a logic or rationality different from the logic in production of goods or administrative work—a rationality of caring—that should be taken into consideration when organizing public care (See Chapter 1). These studies have not had any influence on the planning and political authorities. And, the new educational program for care workers has still not solved the problem of recruiting enough care workers to become a stable workforce in this sector. During the 1980s an increasing bureaucratization and standardization of the services and different organizational reforms took place, and some new occupational education programs for care workers were established. However, lack of recognition and status for frontline care work and for the knowledge and experiences of the care workers continue to be important characteristics of the whole public care system. These characteristics seem immutable. The professionalization of care has implied, first and foremost, better education for administrators and leaders and not for the frontline care workers who are lowest in the hierarchy. Instead, management ideas from the private sector have been taken in by planners and politicians, and these ideas continue to have an increasing influence on public care organizations in all Nordic countries (Vabø 2007).

The 1990s and beyond: the pace of organizational changes and new public management

Public care services for the elderly in the Nordic countries can be said to have been under constant organizational change since these services became part of the welfare state. The pace of change has, however, varied both between countries and over time. During the 1990s it also became evident that changes in ideology take place much more rapidly than changes in everyday practices. Several qualitative studies documented great variation as to how much the *homemaking ideology* still influenced the organizing and practicing of this service. The culture of care can vary even in the same community, as shown by Szebehely (1995), Christensen (1997), and Vabø (2007). At the same time the tendency towards less autonomy and greater subordination in the home helper's job seems to happen everywhere.

An increasing medicalization of the services takes place in all countries as public home care becomes reserved to a greater extent for the most helpless elderly and help with housework becomes a shrinking service. Tasks related to personal care and medical needs have higher prestige than household tasks. This may be one reason why the *disappearance* of housework did not meet much resistance from home helpers as a group, even if it resulted to an increasing extent in them becoming assistants to professional nurses rather than autonomous helpers. The impact of changes in working conditions—greater time pressure and less contact with each client—has, however, been documented. As a result, it becomes increasingly difficult for home helpers to acquire the most satisfying and meaningful aspects of the job, that is, the feeling of giving good care to individuals with whom they become acquainted (Næss and Wærness 1996). The dilemma in their work situation seems to be the same as the dilemma Gough described in her study: 'We are not respected as competent care workers as long as we carry the wash-tub in one hand and support the pensioner with the other. To get recognition for the "invisible" work we are doing, we have to let go of both the wash-tub and the pensioner' (Gough 1987: 212).

Concomitant with the neoliberal turn in welfare policy, a new disciplinary order of managerialism has been imposed on the care workers. This new managerialism has been called *new public management*. Following these new principles of retrenching, rationing, and restructuring care service delivery, the tendency that Eliasson (1992) characterized as the Taylorization of care services has increased during recent years. By Taylorization we mean a horizontal splitting up of the different tasks and an increasing hierarchization of the organization. These processes strengthen the separation of the *work of the hand* and the *work of the head*. This means also that the gap between clients and management has widened. But the increased power of the managers does not necessary mean they have complete or better control than before over the problem of recruiting enough care workers, which takes more and more time resources. Efforts to improve the recruitment situation by educational reforms can easily become a story of failed modernization. The neoliberal ethos has been a legitimating ideology behind setting up a hierarchical task-oriented work culture, which has many of the characteristics of Taylorization: the work that frontline care workers have access to is curtailed by an organization that blurs their work role through an unclear system of task transferrals. At the same time, the system does not value the socially defined care they provide. On the other hand, new individual career opportunities have appeared for the more educated professionals—opportunities not to be better in care work, but to become managers or experts in more specified fields.

A common core finding in a lot of Nordic studies from recent years is that the modernization of the public care services in all the Nordic countries has been on the wrong track for quite a long time now. It is therefore high time to reform the services from the bottom up. One strategy to do this is to build on the knowledge that can be acquired from listening to the yet unheard voices of the care researchers who have tried to analyze these services from such a perspective. Further, reform should build upon the knowledge resources of the experienced frontline workers who may still be found in our public care organizations. For such a long time, diverse management ideas have been sought from other types of work organization in order to make the services *more efficient*. It is high time that the important knowledge resources to be found within the care field come into focus in the planning process. When I say that it is high time, it is because we have good reasons to assume that the proportion of experienced frontline care workers is steadily decreasing. They are substituted by streams of less stable care workers, and this tendency threatens to rapidly exhaust the relevant practical knowledge resources in the field.

Chapter 8
Aiming towards Diversity Welfare in a Global Society

Norio Okazawa

Introduction

Centennial anniversary of diplomatic treaty between Norway and Japan

> People smile and wave their hands from the window—always along the Trondheim canal.

This poem was composed and read by the Japanese Emperor at a New Year Imperial Poetry Reading Party in 2006. His visit to the ancient city of Trondheim in Norway in May 2005, which marked the centennial anniversary of a diplomatic treaty between Norway and Japan, was greatly welcomed by pro-Japan Norwegians.

The King of Norway, Harald V, visited Waseda University in Japan on March 26, 2001. The King was awarded an honorary degree from Waseda University, and he gave a memorial lecture at Okuma Hall, Waseda University. The lecture was titled 'The legacy of Fridtjof Nansen: The devotion for humanitarianism':

> In 1888, at the age of 27, Nansen led his first Arctic Circle expedition. He was very determined to land the east coast of Greenland and made his way on ice across to the west. No one had ever done that before. He continued to advance with the words, 'Go ahead!' This episode tells of his strong determination and 'all or nothing' attitude. Nansen tells later in his book that strong motivation comes from taking the only option available. I would like to remember his words when addressing humanitarian issues.

The King's lecture, with Nansen's words, was very convincing. Nansen was a famous well-rounded Norwegian adventurer whom people admire, and he was also active as a novelist, an athlete, a scientist, a politician, and the first United Nations High Commissioner for Refugees.

The year 2005 was the centennial anniversary of the signing of a treaty of diplomacy between Norway and Japan. The research project that led to this book was planned in this year. I hope our academic exchange continues to develop for the betterment of the welfare system.

Governance in a globalized society

We can find such a case that foreign shareholders complain about and recall the labor negotiations or incentive bonuses at shareholder meetings held at their birthplaces. Numerous highly profitable small companies undertake mergers or acquisitions, and once they become big, administrative functions are relocated to a country with low labor costs.

While small countries try to implement the Kyoto Protocol, the big powers refuse to ratify it. Yet these larger countries have a great responsibility for protecting the global environment. Former United States Vice President Al Gore makes a strong impression on people. He called attention to the need to alleviate poverty and to care for the global environment by attending the 'Live 8' and 'Save Our Selves' concerts and by making the film *An Inconvenient Truth*. Regardless of his title of former Vice President, his influence is not inferior to the current President.

Companies and social movements can cross national borders easily nowadays. State sovereignty was confirmed during the Westphalian sovereignty. However, it now faces the challenge of greatly improved infrastructure for telecommunications and transportation. Not only states, but many kinds of organizations, such as the following, have become actors in governance in globalised society: regional organizations (e.g. the European Union, ASEAN), international organizations (e.g. the United Nations, the G8, UNICEF, the World Health Organization (WHO)), non-governmental organizations (NGOs) and not-for-profit organizations (NPOs) (e.g. Save the Children, the movement against child pornography), local government units that are engaging in international cooperation, large international/multinational firms, and educational research institutions.

A single country is too small to solve problems alone. A century ago approximately forty to fifty countries and regions made up the earth; however, this number has increased to approximately 208. This number does not even include the regions that are moving towards independence. The United Nations has 192 member countries, due perhaps to the existence of many mini/micro countries, which each has a shrinking area of responsibility.

We cannot expect small countries like the Republic of Vanuatu, Andorra, or the Republic of Nauru to solve big policy issues like global warming, desertification, air pollution, or ozone depletion. These issues are even too big for large, strong governments or great economic powers to solve. But at the same time, the state is too big to concern itself with small issues, such as bullying in fundamental schools. We need not use a big power shovel to dig a small hole.

People's desires have increased, and as individual values and lifestyles become more diversified, they require more detailed policy responses. Relatively small issues like establishing local medical systems or selecting building lots for institutions for the elderly are too small for big states to address. Doing so would be a waste of resources. Regional communities or NPOs are more apt at addressing such matters. In a manner of speaking, a huge bulldozer is not required to dig a small hole.

Aim and contents

The aim of this prologue is to introduce the idea of *diversity welfare management* in order to solve the coming challenges in global society.

This prologue has five sections, beginning with this introduction In the second section, 'Lifestyle transition and triggers,' I first analyze changes in society with a theory of games. Second, I show the definition of lifestyle, its component values, and the life stages where the values are selectively put. The life stages here include childhood, youth, adulthood, old age, and so on. I show that peoples' sense of value depends on the life stage, and I also show some reasons for the diversity of lifestyle.

The third section, 'Changes in working styles and challenges in Japan,' describes changes in working styles and their reasons. This section focuses many current challenges of the labor market in Japan.

The fourth section, 'Idea of diversity welfare management as a policy object,' illustrates the necessity to set up and maintain sustainable sefety-net. I show the important aspect of how to politically meet the needs for a diversified form of welfare.

Finally, the conclusion follows. Governance in a globalised society, nation-states, and decentralization can be either a force for secession or integration—a reason for competition or a seedbed for cooperation. 'Open up, open up, and open up even more'—this should be the attitude of government towards managing diversity. Open up and share more information, and expand the opportunity to participate and consider. This can specifically be in regard to public services such as child care and elderly care, educational services to catch up on current information and technology, and job training for new skills and easy transfer for all people. It seems that there is no other way than what is mentioned above to manage diversity under a parliamentary democracy. Society is ever-changing and we never know what the future will bring. Parliamentary democracy tries to gather everyone's suggestions to address problems. Authority and justice in decision making only develops people's understanding. The more consensus it can bring, the more burden people could bear. The welfare society can develop together with democracy.

Lifestyle transition and triggers

Components of lifestyle and transition of society

Lifestyle narrowly defines how an individual lives; it is the incorporation of values that one emphasizes in choices and decisions and to some extent it is what an individual likes and tries to realize to some degree in the duration of life. The choice of lifestyle depends on choice and priority of values, and how people work to realize values. Ways of realizing values and how much people work for it are two important factors. In this context, values refer to what one wants now and always. Values can be power, authority, wealth or other financial strength, honor, publicity, specific technology and information, knowledge, health, family, social activity, respect, and love (Shigeru 1996: 1–4).

Fundamental values like these are limited in resources (sometimes in budget), and the sum total that the actor gains as a profit is already determined. It is like a fixed-sum game. Here *game* means that actors try to gain some values from resources. If the number of actors who want to gain a profit increases, the competition becomes harder in such a fixed-sum game. The game would be most competitive if actors try to gain authority, land, or sovereignty. It is a zero-sum game. In this game-situation, what is gained by the winner is lost by the loser. The total sum of all players' pay-off is always zero. There is no possibility of peaceful co-existence. It is a most merciless game.

However, most of the values people pursue in order to be happy are based on resources gained through the process by which human beings develop nature—the land, the sea, the sky, the ocean bed, or the universe. Throughout history technology has helped us increase value-options to be happy. This is a moderate competition and resources are shared by self-help efforts and allocated as variable-sum games. Scientific technology has accelerated the speed of the competition.

But these resources are not considered to be part of a variable-sum game. New actors such as new industrial countries also participated in the competitive market, with a desire to industrialize these resources. This effort required enormous resources, and it began to be recognized that oil, gas, iron, and food were limited in their reserves. What was once believed to be allocated as a variable-sum game assumed the features of a zero-sum game.

The more competitive allocation becomes, the greater the amount of funds required to procure basic resources. One cannot avoid social disparity, unless one controls one's desire to a certain level or expects scientific development to gain more resources.

We can find some countries that care about the environment—for example, where excrement is used to fuel buses, or where geothermal energy is used to heat water. Some countries have developed wind power as their major export industry, and some countries develop and use alternative forms of energy from resources such as wood or from recycling.

The social axiom on this globe is equal opportunity. No country can deny the industrialization of another. Social responsibility within developed countries requires proactive investment in technology to develop new resources. They must improve conventional technology related to the five Rs—refuse, reuse, re-birth, reduce, and recycle. Welfare governance in the twenty-first century starts here. Global leaders must start dealing with, and give priority preference to, global issues before economics, labor, or welfare.

Next I look at the lifestyle components stages. There are turning points in one's life, where structural or functional features of the stages define an individual by his/her lifestyle characteristics. Life does not develop solely on its own but is influenced by circumstances and relationships. How does the current global environment change lifestyle stages? How would an individual map his/her life then? The lifestyle stages are:

Stage 1: life delivered: conception, start life (birth)
Stage 2: raised: grow up at home and in a community
Stage 3: learn (at home, at school, in a community)
Stage 4: graduate (compulsory education), advanced education
Stage 5: work: employed
Stage 6: fall in love: meeting, relationship, separation
Stage 7: marry: marriage, living together
Stage 8: deliver life: (first child, second child, third child, etc.)
Stage 9: childrearing (at home, in the nursery, and in community) and education (high school, postgraduate, lifelong learning) and vocational education and return to working
Stage 10: turning point: job leaving, unemployment, job change, job training and re-employment; divorce and remarriage; severe illness and struggle with disease and return to work

Stage 11: children become independent, children marry, grandchildren born
Stage 12: retired: retirement from work, post-retirement life, pension starts
Stage 13: rest, heal: ill, long-term care, bedridden
Stage 14: separation: partner's bereavement, back to single life again
Stage 15: die: death, in grave.

Trigger to diversification—environmental challenge and lifestyle change

Since late in the twentieth century, many industrial countries have been processing structural reform against new environmental challenges in politics, economics, and the social system. The challenges are as follows: (1) low birthrates/more elderly, (2) globalization, (3) rapid innovations in information and transportation technology, and (4) environmental degradation. These challenges could have a dramatic affect on the way we live. The scale and the speed of changes are quite different among countries, but there is also similarity. This is inevitable in any system.

Low birthrate and more elderly

If a human being has a lifespan of eighty-five years, then he/she has a total of 744,600 hours, while 120 years ago, he/she would have had 385,440 hours in an average lifespan of forty-four years. A difference of 359,160 hours has increased equally for an individual as their fundamental resource. Lifestyles have changed and one can now experience more; however, these experiences can be both positive and negative. The matters we worry about never go away and our lifestyles will become different as we gain more time as we become older.

The arrival of aged society and longer life expectancy change our lifestyles fundamentally. Many developed countries are trying to promote fewer working hours and more holidays, and are encouraging people to use this time. With one's lifespan increasing, the total number of hours one works accounts for less time in one's life and more leisure time is available. People will be motivated to try different activities in order to make the most out of life.

In a community of the elderly, for instance, volunteer work might be popular. Learning opportunities and methods of communicating might be different, as well. Fewer working hours and more leisure time might motivate us to undertake self-development and self-discovery and our styles of work might also change.

The style of our working life will also change. More senior people will move into the labor market. There will be more people who will not dedicate themselves to the same role in a single company; rather, changing jobs will be more common, which will in turn change business management itself.

The conventional Japanese business model has been characterized as follows: lifetime employment, a seniority-based wage system, and an in-company union. This model also has a custom whereby companies employ new people at the same time every year, and every company has a bonus system. This Japanese business model once expected a low-cost labor force that continuously participated in working for its businesses. A low birthrate has, however, negatively affected business.

In 2006 Japan had 1.06 million newborns, in contrast to 2.70 million in 1947. The current labor force still expects lifetime employment and a seniority-based wage system, while the younger, less experienced labor force receives less. How can we sustain global competition? A new business management is required, but it is not easy to put this into practice.

In addition, due to decreasing birthrates, the size of the family has shrunk in size from a traditionally large one and has changed its social function. In the past, the family had the following functions: a sexual function, a reproductive function, a childrearing function, a social function, an economic/productive function, an economic/consuming function, an educational function, a protective/caring/nursing/helping function, an entertainment function, a rest and comfort-giving function, a religious/ceremonial function, a position-giving function, and a judging/penalty-giving function. The birthrate is declining more rapidly than ever and due to its decline most of these functions are dysfunctional and no longer work. What other alternatives exist?

Globalization

Globalization has developed through many factors—for example, traveling overseas, establishing international relationships/marriages, working on long-term overseas assignments, studying abroad, living in foreign countries, having diverse colleagues around the world, and being overseas pensioners. These factors make us aware of global issues, as well. People would never realize the significance of matters in the world without being aware of national borders and having the actual experience of interacting overseas. Global issues cannot be solved by the principle of competition, and they become more serious as globalization develops. One nation-state cannot solve such matters on its own. The current severe global environment and the above issues require a global welfare system that can be applied across borders.

Rapid innovation in information and transportation technology

Advanced information technology is challenging the conventional lifestyle. More people are working at home and online, and there is more flexibility in working hours and more diversity in company strategy and organization. There is no need to locate a production site in a big city. Business is becoming *borderless*. Many of the basic economics have been overturned by the rapid innovation in information and transportation technology.

If a small incident occurs somewhere in the world, it can be broadcast around the world within a minute. There are more opportunities to join in the new global coalition. Other variables have also influenced our lifestyles, such as the washing machine, the vacuum cleaner, the microwave, the dishwasher, the large refrigerator, high-speed flight, the computer, and the mobile telephone. Without the invention of these technologies, more women could not have gone to work. This type of historical perspective in science and technology will be an important analytic framework when people analyze the northern European welfare state, in which science and technology are important factors.

Environmental degradation

We are now facing a situation in which we must pay the costs of mass production, distribution, consumption, and disposal. These issues are similar to global warming, desertification problems, abnormal climate change, air pollution, noise pollution, ozone depletion, and depleted natural resources. It seems that these environmental challenges are a warning to the conceited scientific technology—or an unexpected new frontier to them. As the global environment worsens, more welfare issues are created. People's ways of life, food, holidays, and retirement are influenced. Changes to the global environment could produce unexpected welfare issues.

Changes in working styles and challenges in Japan

International migration of labor

A diversified lifestyle includes domestic and global travel. A competitor can exist in the domestic local community, as well as in the global community. The improvement of transportation infrastructure has reduced physical distance and the improvement of communication infrastructure could bridge the gap that people feel. A person has access to the world from his/her living room, study, office, or from a restaurant. World information is widely available, with more options, and one can obtain enough information, along with various options to consider, before putting a plan into action.

In lifelong learning there are *learning emigrants*, *education emigrants* (such as researchers and teachers), *labor emigrants* (such as workers who wish to challenge their talents and abilities), *executive emigrants*, and *management emigrants*, who desire better locations for their businesses. All of these people travel globally. A *worker* or *sport player emigrant* could be included here, as well, if his/her achievement for the same workload is not valued in one place. A *tax emigrant* may be a company that wishes to relocate for tax purposes. A *pension emigrant* is the pensioner who moves to another country because his/her pension is not enough in his/her own country due to inflation. An *environmental emigrant* is a person who is more concerned about his/her health. There are many cases in which people relocate overseas due to their tiny houses or the traffic in their home countries. A *post-retirement emigrant* wishes to have a different life after retirement and may stay overseas for a long period. If one relocates to a location with better welfare resources, he/she will be a *welfare emigrant* or a *medical service emigrant*. A *cultural emigrant* is attracted to the history, town, art, and traditional craft in that country to which he/she moves.

Competition begins domestically and globally in many social sectors, from the education industry to the service industry for pensioners. How do companies and unions manage this diversification? Diversified values should be applied at first in the decision-making process. The more diversified the employment system becomes, the more options it makes available to us in life. This is the standard condition for the *society diversified in its working style*. More social disparity might be corrected and structured there, but a mature society will not conduct unreasonable restructuring to lay off people or require excess work in the name of *diversity in working style*.

Competition in the global market will become more serious. In these situations the labor market will continue to become diversified and flexible. Diversity and flexibility in the labor market will require a mature society, which corresponds to new challenges there. Global telecommunications networks will also help the process of diversification. An advanced industrial society will require company ethics to uphold *fair trade* and *fair work* regulations.

The labor market, people's style of work, and the employment system are obviously going to become diversified. Thus there will be many new styles of working and living; for instance, full-time work/employment, temporary work/employment, contract work/employment, part-time work/employment, regularly based new employment, mid-career employment, easy means of changing jobs or taking early retirement, no employment for young people, NEET[1] (young people Not in Education, Employment, or Training), domestic work for international companies, work overseas for domestic companies, work overseas for international companies, businesses at home/overseas, *Hikikomori*,[2] *Sotokomori*,[3] work contracts on an annual salary system, work at home, a SOHO[4] (Small Office Home Office) style that involves working closely with the internet, and telework.

The infrastructure for telecommunications and transportation is still improving. People can work at home and from a distance. People outside the country can also engage in work. In the near future, a new lifestyle will be more widespread. People can choose to work in the city/at home and have a family or live in the suburbs/overseas. These options can, of course, be reversed.

The rate of second-home ownership is one measurement that indicates the maturity of the welfare system in an economy. The ownership rate can be increased, of course, by reducing laborers' working time and by laborers taking more holidays.

People have chosen where to live based on where they work. We can say that people have not been comfortable at home because they have to choose a place of residence with consideration given to overtime work. It means that people have to stay in towns where they are able to go home even late at night.

Improvement in the infrastructure for telecommunications and transportation will give us new lifestyles with more available options in the area where we work and live. This lifestyle diversity will yield a broader range of values and encourage society to be more diversified.

The fluctuations in traditional organizations in Japan

Economic globalization cannot be avoided. A small country should not be bothered by global matters. Each country should find its own way to provide benefits for its citizens. International competition will emerge when energy sources or raw materials, such as iron, pulp, and cement, become limited. A small country cannot help but enter into such competition. Oils, raw materials, or foods can be the basis for competition among those who strongly depend on these resources. Unless such goods are produced domestically, they must be procured on the global market. A country with a large population that desires to live like the G7 nations will try and catch up to their standards. The principle of equal opportunity is applied in this global society. There should be tips for us to learn from cases in which small countries maintain a competitive position in international markets.

The conventional Japanese business characteristics are lifetime employment, a seniority-based wage system, an in-company union, vast numbers of new employees begin their career on the 1st April, and bonuses paid simultaneously, in principle on July and December, to all workers. People can commit their lives to the company under a long-term contract. Traditionally and fundamentally, even now in the big organizations, job training was conducted in-company, and the employee was trained in the necessary skills. A salary was paid according to individual needs, so each employee could receive the necessary pay at the necessary time.

A company treated an employee as a family member, and therefore the employee had no doubts about committing his/her life to the company; however, this conventional management style now no longer seems attractive to people. The level of welfare in the company is considered too low.

First, there is neither gender equality nor equal opportunity in these traditional business structures. Gender roles seem to be more stable in the more conventional management style. Such companies still believe in *men at work, women at home*, and assign roles or positions based on this belief. The *opportunity cost* for women is too high, especially during the maternity period and raising a child. Maternity leave is short, and income is reduced.

Second, a seniority-based wage system can function unequally for employees who have different needs from other people. For instance, a young employee who originally planned to stay or who stayed only five years at one company might leave before his/her raise in pay. He/she might not have been paid enough for his/her performance. How could he/she be patient with his/her manager, who is most probably unqualified and not motivated enough, but who receives a high salary? A key human resource is not used properly under the seniority-based wage system that requires everyone to work in the same manner.

Third, those who cannot accept the family-like culture might be forced to sacrifice themselves. They cannot refuse to work extra hours, during holidays, and even without pay as *service overtime work*. Some companies require their employees to work unpaid overtime at home. Overtime work is required regularly, and employees are required to be organization men/women and workaholics. They cannot ask for a day off, although such instances may happen once in a while, and more than 50% of holidays remain untaken at the end of the year. Moreover, it is impossible to take a three- to four-week holiday. Long working hours make it difficult to make time for other important duties or occasions such as holidays, education, raising children, housekeeping, or socializing.

The purpose of life is not just to work, and people's values are not defined only by their work performances. Diversified values are desired in society. Companies are beginning to support the balance of work and family, but this is just the beginning. Over the long term, it will benefit companies and unions to attract and motivate good people who can perform productively. People are motivated when satisfied with their work and other social activities, not just with financial rewards or career advancement.

Fourth, the conventional organization hires many employees at once for lifetime employment, so they can start work at the same time. Professionals who join or leave midway might be treated differently. Promotion is normally awarded earlier and an external training workshop is given preferentially to the full-time employee who has worked over the years. There is a logic that distinguishes *internal* and *external* employees. An organization should be more open to its people and their opportunities. A conventional organization does not respond properly to the diversified requests from its employees, with their various environmental challenges and diversified lifestyles. Women, senior people, foreigners, or the disabled all look for opportunities to work at each life stage, but their talents are currently being wasted. Candidates are often rejected only because of their age, while employers ignore all of their positive attributes and their good attitudes. The traditional Japanese organization now requires adjustments that take into account environmental changes. This is currently the transition period, when we cannot see exactly what the next organization will be like.

Diversity welfare management as a policy object

The policy object is now to improve people's lives so they can feel secure and live safely. This means that people do not need to panic when something unexpected happens. In addition, the unexpected should not occur too often, or if it does, people can deal with it through the options available to them. In order to make that happen, as summarized, we set up a welfare system called a *safety net* that we can maintain; we must foster and develop an internationally competitive industry, as 'powerful industry is the indispensable fuel for welfare' and for the stable and peaceful labor market, and we ensure employment to keep people away from the risk of unemployment.

Set up and enhance the safety net—eliminate the fear

First of all, security and safety must be institutionalized. People feel anxious when they do not know what the future might bring and are unsure of how to deal with it.

Economic power has taken advantage of this anxiety and fear in order to become competitive and motivated until it showed a path of geometric growth. We had to turn anxiety and fear into competing energy and then into the motivation for growth. Both education and work have emphasized that one must 'do it, otherwise...,' 'study hard, otherwise...,' 'work hard, otherwise...,' 'save money, otherwise...' People have studied hard, worked hard, and saved money for fear of an uncertain future and panic at the unexpected. Careerism has justified working overtime, on holidays, without pay. Employees were always at risk of sudden death or death due to overwork. Such dedication also appeared to be competition to show company loyalty.

Some other anxieties are related to disease, unemployment, aging, loss of educational opportunities, social isolation, giving birth/experiencing infertility, manmade disasters such as fires or car accidents, death by natural disaster (e.g. a typhoon or an earthquake), and loss of living space due to global warming or the problem of desertification.

One of the worst forms of anxiety would be looking for a job after losing one. In a competitive global market, the manufacturing sector is transferred to a low-wage country at first, but the nonmanufacturing sector or the back office will eventually follow that trend as well. Optic fiber technology is creating a new revolution for working styles.

Blue-collar work, as well as white-collar work, will compete in a low-wage labor country. The launching of more satellites and the expansion of airline service networks give us faster access worldwide, and technology supports the labor network. People with postgraduate degrees in business can return to their home countries and train others. Low-wage labor can replace not only the manufacturing sector but also the nonmanufacturing sector or the back office through the information technology/digital revolution.

This kind of transfer/replacement can be accomplished easily, without degrading the quality of management. More countries oriented towards marketing can set up safety nets sooner, because they will recognize the negative effects of globalization. Otherwise, organizations cannot even start their internal reforms.

It is essential to set up safety nets and educational environments (learning, training, and re-education). Good public services should also be provided in case something unexpected happens. People's anxiety can be removed not only by providing opportunities for re-education but by offering unemployment insurance, health insurance, pensions, and welfare benefits.

In some countries a good balance remains between a high standard of welfare and international competitiveness. It is only a matter of agreement if people are happy to pay their taxes to buy security in society (Rengoh sohgo seikatsukaihatsu kenkyujo 2007: 87, 93).

Making policy for *extra* time, space, goods, money, and relaxation

Removing anxiety does not make people feel entirely safe. People cannot necessarily deal with issues spontaneously when they occur. They might just wish they had some *extra* time, space, goods, and money, and feel like they could then have extra space to relax.

Regarding money, the following issues must be worked upon first: the *working poor*, an appropriate minimum wage, and an appropriate wage for nonpermanent employees.

The issue regarding space is quite serious. More and more institutions for the elderly are being built, but we have to be more creative in the locations and the living spaces of these establishments.

What is the most important policy objective in the governance of welfare? Should we ever let the elderly be bedridden? Or should we try our hardest to avoid the elderly being bedridden? And should we invest less in nursing care but more on the universal design for a national land plan and in rehabilitation institutions?

Another option, given that some bedridden elderly cannot be avoided and we invest greatly on nursing care for them, is to at least make institutions accessible. This is one of the most important discussion points regarding welfare governance as birthrates decline and the numbers of senior people rise.

Regarding goods to make our lives easier, we need to ensure that support devices and facilities for nursing care are more accessible and obtainable. Great numbers of excellent new devices or facilities are currently being developed, but are not actually being introduced to institutions due to the costly reconstruction work required, so the hard work of care workers is not being eased and institutions cannot be constantly monitored. The minimum wage of care workers is unbelievably low and institutions protect their inside information from outsiders.

Caring for a support person is as important as caring for those who require nursing care. Nursing care is characterized as low-wage and hard work. It is difficult to clearly define each job assignment, and sometimes the employee receives no compensation, no limitation on his/her duties, or is required to work twenty-four-hour shifts. Caring for a support person should be the first priority in welfare governance in the twenty-first century.

Better living environments for daily life

It should be verified whether the following living spaces are secure and safe: living space (e.g. accessibility); commuting space and transportation (e.g. the sidewalk/street is distinct, and there is a universal design for each train station); work space and office space (e.g. is it spacious enough to be comfortable, do individuals have their own rooms?); leisure/learning space (e.g. group lessons); socializing/communication space; social activity space (e.g. for NPO activity); medical/rest/treatment space (e.g. from group room to individual room); and environmental space.

The work space especially remains to be improved. People spend a third of each day at work, so it is absolutely important to make sure it is secure and safe. Medical/treatment space is also important and cannot be ignored; often these types of facilities vary considerably in quality.

A composite approach should be taken in considering the relationship between *living space* and those who actually live there. For instance, take *living environment*, which concerns foreigners living in Japan or Japanese living overseas, and consider the above eight parameters from a senior person's perspective. They are faced with the same kind of welfare needs. *Living space* and *living actor* would sum up so many parameters but we must consider the best ways from the perspective of resource administration and management.

Ability of choice in many options

The more diversified a society is in its values, the more options exist for individual lifestyles and work. Each individual desires to select and make decisions on his/her own from a variety of life courses. However, it is a totally different issue to have many options and to enjoy them equally. The following will be important: whether the individual can make choices by him- or herself; an increasing number of options should be available; available options should be expanded; and one should keep refining the ability to choose.

While many options are presently available, *self-organization* is defined as a person's ability to select and decide on a life course based on his/her own values, to invest him- or herself in the chosen life course, and to continue to pursue it at his/her own risk. A tough and sustainable welfare society needs many such self-organized people in solidarity, otherwise it cannot sustain itself.

A tough society can take appropriate action, even when something unusual happen. Equality and equal opportunity are what support self-organized people. It is especially important for us to provide them with an information network and a lifelong learning opportunity.

Highly taxed society and solidarity

Low birthrates and an aging society are rapidly spreading, and these phenomena are challenging conventional commonsense. These trends will also change the lifestyles of single people, and the styles of relationships, marriages, births, childrearing, and nursing care.

More improvement in welfare would inevitably impose greater tax burdens on us. The total amount of working time for the individual, however, does not extend as far as the rise in life expectancy. There is a limit to how long people can actually work.

A payable tax burden is limited. People must be kept highly motivated if the government is to ask for greater tax burdens. In that process, the government might be forced to admit the inappropriate means it has conventionally used. A flexible method can apply to solve multiple issues. A flexible technique can allocate help to the public or individuals or both together under the current situation. The Scandinavian countries have proactively taken a flexible approach to change within the labor market. These five countries together have a total of twenty-four million people. In contrast, senior Japanese people are expected to number 34.7 million in 2028. Their welfare policy has laid down a foundation for the work-sharing idea.

In Japan 1.5 people will work in 2050 to support the pension for each senior person, while 12.1 people worked towards that goal in 1950. Numerous issues still exist: pensions, health insurance, nursing care insurance, employment insurance, labor insurance, and welfare public assistance. The increase in such burdens cannot be avoided. There is no way to reduce the burden on people unless we have a larger labor force or more taxpayers.

In the process of solving some environmental challenges, universal solidarity is required, as well as solidarity among men and women, among the different generations, and within the regional community.

Universal solidarity is obviously necessary to solve some environmental challenges. Japan is highly dependent on imports for energy and material resources and food. Ensuring a regular procurement route will be a lifeline, since most Japanese trade is processing trade. A decline in international competitiveness would make it difficult to procure welfare and financial resources. As a country that lacks resources, Japan must ensure it has the trust of the international society. The Scandinavian countries proactively accept refugees, and the high amount of official development assistance for each individual demonstrates the countries' high credibility in international society. With a favorable public image and technological development, they maintain great international competitiveness. This initiative was perhaps taken in spite of the limited capability of one nation's welfare. Their significant interest in fair trade and fair work also indicates the same initiative. In any case, welfare resources or human resources are both procured on the international competitive market. When we see such an environment, *global welfare governance* is necessary for the present society.

Solidarity among regional communities and generations is also necessary. A government cannot explain the validity of the welfare system if there is disparity of burden and benefit among regional communities or generations. Pensions and other welfare policies go through the process of exchanging burden for benefit from a long-term perspective. *Sustainability* will be the important element in this. Future generations are absolutely the stakeholders for welfare policies, with their importance increasing over time. They might resist participating in welfare policy unless the present generations pay the social costs for the future generation. The gross domestic product (GDP) of Japan is almost 500 trillion yen, and total debt is around 800 trillion yen. The national budget is 83 trillion yen. Everyone, including new-born infants, borrows six million yen. The average annual wage of a private institution is about 4.5 million yen. How can such a huge debt be paid back by the coming generations? Unless we prove *sustainability*, we cannot connect the different generations through trust. Intergenerational solidarity is necessary in societies with heavier burdens. This explains why an active labor market policy focuses on the younger generations.

Regional disparities are often seen in medical/nursing care/welfare institutions, the aging rate, the budget scale, the population, job numbers, volunteer numbers, and infrastructure development. A government subsidy system should be set up to automatically calculate a balanced ratio of security and safety without being affected by differences in population. Fairness of generations should also be balanced for burdens and benefits because there is a time lag between when burdens and entitlements such as a pension system start. Thirty years seems enough time to initiate change in people's values and lifestyles. A government subsidy system should comply with a fair standard to convince participants beyond a timeframe of thirty years. It is too great a change in society to estimate people's life plans in thirty year's time and to start payment of premiums. High moral values of leaders (such as those in politics, government, economics, or justice) are more important requirements in order to encourage intergenerational solidarity and to improve the validity of the system. Moral values are required the most among leaders in welfare governance in order to manage the limited natural resources of the actors. This is proved by the fact that any small impropriety will be held liable in welfare society. The top leaders in each field should be selected from people aged forty-five to fifty-five years, so that they have enough time to make up for losses if failure occurs.

Regarding the solidarity between men and women, both should start to participate in the following at once: for men, housekeeping, childrearing, and nursing care; and, for women, the labor market. One breakthrough will be to reduce working hours and to enable employees to take holidays. The Japan labor environment still has issues in its rising numbers of nonpermanent workers, women's working conditions, and long working hours, and especially *service overtime*, which is seen in many workplaces. Thirty percent of part-time workers are said to work overtime as *service* without pay (Asahi Shimbun 2006).

Conclusion

The start: reduce working hours

What kind of economic power is it, where people work overtime without question and 10% work until eleven o'clock at night (Rengoh sohgo seikatsukaihatsu kenkyujo 2007: 35)? There are no limits to working overtime—this tendency is obviously one of the biggest reasons why employees are deprived of time to relax and also to participate in housework and childrearing. Excessive work can kill people suddenly. People are pressured not to refuse such work, and say, 'I have worked like hell,' 'I will work until I die' (Morioka 2006). I actually know of such cases and want to give this message to the next generation.

The work–life balance cannot use the excuse of diversity to make people work excessive overtime, to be inappropriately or lowly paid, to work on limited contracts, or to work unlimited hours, even at the risk of their health. It is impossible to reduce working hours in a work place with a culture in which people are always concerned to agree with others.

The reduction of working hour is a point of departure. In 1988 the government set numeric targets to reduce working time to 1800 hours a year as an economic management policy objective. The target was not easily met.

While some people work excessively and fear dying from hard work (or too much work), others hold no work position and, in contrast, are suffering severe distress at being excluded. In Japan more than 30,000 people commit suicide every year (32,249 during 2008). The goal of 1800 hours is calculated based on working no overtime and using paid leave completely. However, the actual time spent as overtime work is reported to be around 2100 hours, and only 45% to 55% (at a maximum) of paid holidays are taken, which is about ten days per year. Most holidays are never taken in full.

Realize diversity welfare management

The twentieth century saw many developments in transportation/communication technology, production/logistics, medical and nursing care/support/equipment (including life-support measures), habilitation and rehabilitation—and we cannot ignore globalization, the aging society, the global population expansion, or a broader living space.

Information and consumer goods easily travel around the globe, and people's desires spread worldwide. Technology or natural resources are only obtainable through competition. The more that options in society become diversified, the more diversified our lifestyles become. This also leads to disparities due to the wide range of options. Do these options represent lifeblood for new life, or another form of anxiety?

Organizations and society must be flexible regarding the current situation, and must strike the right balance. It is not reasonable to try to adjust every conventional custom or rule to fit the present.

The *unexpected* will easily become the *expected* in a society in which things always change. Job positions have been considerably modified, deleted, or added. Management in an organization or society has so many factors to consider: gender, age, educational background, income group, nationality, ethnicity, citizenship, type of visa, technology, qualification, employment style, and location. We have already arrived at global personnel administration.

The present age requires diversity management to control both an organization and society. Diversity is required not only in a service provider but also in a recipient and in welfare services. Welfare governance in the twenty-first century aims to establish the concept of welfare governance at a global level from a diversity management perspective.

Diversity requires flexibility as its best partner. When discussing public service and social welfare, it tends to focus only on controlling the welfare budget. There will be some debate about *limited government* and eliminating benefits.

Yet several countries have much greater authority as large governments and still maintain their budget surpluses. In such countries people enjoy universal public services with higher taxes, and the governments have core policies to provide universal services based on solidarity and they can cope well with changes of society flexibly.

Industrial welfare is judged fairly. Welfare is a huge market to which governments devote an enormous amount of public funds. Governments account for services evenly, expecting to have financial effects or employment inducements, and try to modify the market against diversity.

There is an interesting case about a *patient hotel* in Sweden—a hospital that uses vacant rooms as hotel accommodation. The process focuses on how to provide welfare services and how to advance reform—the public institution is made private, regulations are reduced, and the bureaucratic structure is reformed. The idea of running a hotel at a hospital contributes to the debate about limited government and fiscal health, about how to interact with the government, and how to create and maintain employment. Medical services are consistent, and the case noted above is a proactive use of a dormant resource after strict cost calculation. 'Adjusting three sides of welfare, finance, and industry' is an important viewpoint, considering people are reluctant to bear the burdens (Miyazawa 2006). People understand the decision because it is a flexible challenge in the direction of new diversity, not a compromise with reality.

How do we meet the consumer's need for diversified welfare? The expectation for the welfare stakeholder expands greatly towards environmental challenges. The Scandinavian countries have taken enormous responsibility, deploying a wide safety net, and have invested taxes as a policy. They are now trying to find ways to move towards diversification in the face of revolution as a free choice.

The public sector was downsized first in the non-welfare field and then selectively in the welfare sector, while avoiding an extreme decline in service levels. Governments pursued new recruitment possibilities, prevented a decline in service levels, and expanded options. At the same time, an active labor market policy was implemented, because ensuring employment and minimizing social disparity ensures the sustainability of the safety net. A preferential policy objective is now set to maintain an unemployment rate of 3%, which is the full employment level, enhancing the consumer's independent management skill and empowerment. Rather than being insecure and fearful, security and safety enable a society to grow as a great economic system, with GDP over $25,000 per capita, like Scandinavian countries.

Notes

Chapter 1

1 This chapter was first published as an article in the journal *Economic and Industrial Democracy*, 1984, pp. 185–212.
2 On the basis of the evidence from social policy research, it seems unlikely that such a change will take place in the Scandinavian countries, at least in the short run.
3 Two surveys based on random samples of old people (70+) in the same Norwegian municipality in 1969 and 1981 show this to be the case for care in old age. In 1969 16% of the aged preferred public care over family care, while this proportion had increased to 58% in 1981 (Daatland 1983).
4 The most well-known feminist analyses on the first phase of the new women's movement focused mainly on the exploitative nature of women's traditional roles (de Beauvoir 1953; Friedan 1963; Firestone 1971; Millett 1971; Mitchell 1971). More recently, however, feminist writers working from their experiences in this new movement have struggled to redefine the possible grounds of feminist theory. This has also led to refocusing on positive experiences of traditional care giving in the private sphere, especially on the experiences of motherhood (Smith 1979; Friedan 1981; O'Brien 1981). One reason for the need for these new kinds of analyses could be that analyses like de Beauvoir's and Firestone's create visions of a future society that most women probably do not want to see realized. For a woman to be liberated, she must not, according to de Beauvoir, give birth. Firestone has the vision of a society where biological reproduction no longer takes place, but has been substituted by technological means for totally mechanistic reproduction.
5 In the social policy debate on more *informal care*, most often no clear distinction is made between *self-care* and *caring for others*. These two concepts are, however, related to the contradictory values of independence and self-sufficiency on the one hand, and the values of responsibility and consideration for *others'* wellbeing on the other. A clear distinction between them is necessary to make visible that these values often give rise

to quite opposite priorities, both in everyday life and in the distribution of scarce resources for public care.

6 In the guidance literature published around the turn of the century for both wives and nurses, we find explicit advice on how they should behave in such situations. Most often women are strongly recommended to obey the husband or the doctor.

7 As we do not know to what extent women's practices have changed according to the changes in the experts' advice, historical studies tell most about changes in ideology. In the field of obstetrics, however, we have hard data on deaths attributed to puerperal fever and on infant mortality rates, which clearly show that the conversion from midwife to doctor at various points in time heightened the risk of death both for mothers and children. See, for instance, Branca (1975: 74–112).

8 The public discussion about the need for parents' education is not today, as in former times, related to problems of physical care, but to problems of bettering the psycho-social conditions for children's development. How to organize such education without professionalizing the socialization process, and without disabling the parents in the attempt to support them, is admitted to be a problem. See, for instance, 'Psychosocial conditions for development in early childhood' (1973).

9 Holter et al. (1967) found that housewives' actual need for information was greatest on topics related to children's development. In general, the expressed need for information was highest among the most educated housewives and in the most urbanized districts. Oakley (1974) finds the social context in which the role of the mother is carried out today very dissatisfactory, as social isolation and constant responsibility are general problems for modern mothers of all classes in urban communities.

10 Dawe argues that one important reason that Weber gave analytic primacy to the instrumentally rational action was the scientific aspiration he brought to sociology. As such action was crucially concerned with the scientifically accurate relationship between means and ends, it was the most easily understandable and explicable type in the rigorous and exact terms scientific analysis demanded. Thus, even if Weber acknowledges that actual social actions and relationships manifest various combinations of elements of all his types of actions and orientations, he does not analyze them in this way; i.e. for the various ways in which they manifest such combinations. Instead, the instrumentally rational action became the yardstick for analyses of actual courses of action, which were viewed in terms of their approximation to or deviation from it. Dawe argues that for sociological analysis in general, the resort to science leads to a denial of

human agency. To respect and grasp and articulate the essential autonomy, contingency, and creativity of human agency, sociology, in Dawe's opinion, must abandon its obsolete and imperious scientific pretension, 'which cuts us off from the world of which we also are members' (Dawe 1978: 409). Instead, Dawe suggests another metaphor for sociology other than science: the metaphor of conversation.

11 Russell Hochschild (1975: 299–300) argues that the image of the sentient actor makes us attentive to the fact that the *social* goes deeper than our current images of the social actor have led us to suppose. Roles and relations are surely not social patterns that apply only to thought and action, leaving feeling an untouched, timeless, and universal constant. We therefore should integrate the sociology of the head with the sociology of the heart.

12 For someone who has not learned to cook, however, this is not obvious, and in general most of us very often forget how much learning is required even for what may seem to be the simplest tasks.

13 In Sweden a special formal training for home helps has been organized by many municipalities in order to increase the supply of home helps. So far, these training programs have not been very successful. A very high proportion of the women who have done this training say that the actual content in the job does not correspond very well to the expectations they got from training, and that they therefore want other types of jobs (*Pensionärundersökningens rapporter om social hemhjälp m.m.* 1979: 47–51).

14 Ve (1982) shows how 'the hidden curriculum' in the whole educational system furthers instrumentalism at the sacrifice of the expressive. Apart from the first years in school, where there is some room for the giving of care to each other according to his/her personal needs, the school mainly conveys values connected to instrumentalism. As it is not made visible how this value-orientation conflicts with the rationality of caring, this created special problems for girls, especially from the working class.

15 This class difference among women is related to the descriptions of class differences in general. Researchers disagree in their interpretations of the working-class lifestyle but many have pointed out the greater tendency to expressiveness compared with the middle class (e.g. Bernstein 1975; Sennett and Cobb 1972). To bring sociology closer to the realities both of the working class and to women, we should cease to treat instrumentality and expressiveness (or rationality and emotionality) as two mutually exclusive qualities of action and should instead treat them as separate continua that vary independently and can be applied to a single action.

16 See Gullestad (1984). The importance of the care-giving work of nannies and maids for children in the higher classes is nearly invisible in the research literature. Freud, for instance, when discussing the relation between mother, father, and child, did not problematize very much what children's relations to nannies and servants could mean. As most of Freud's patients came from bourgeois or upper-class households, we can assume that in early childhood they were mostly taken care of by servants.

17 This statement was given at a seminar for representatives of different voluntary organizations and of the Ministry of Health and Social Affairs in Norway in 1976. In the published report from this seminar, no one expressed any objection to this view.

18 These figures are given by Levin and Idler (1981: 259) without rendering any account of how they are calculated. In documents from the World Health Organization not formally published, I found the same figures.

Chapter 2

1 This chapter is a revised version of my article 'The modernisation of power in Norwegian home care services.' The detailed discussion of changing power structures within this original article is replaced by comparisons with Japanese elderly care and by an extended modernisation perspective. Thanks to Kari Wærness at the University in Bergen and Doria Pilling at City University in London for useful comments.

2 The facts about Japan are from information about 'The Care for the Elderly in Sweden and in Japan,' no. 4, February 9, 2007 (*http://www.wao.or.jp/yamanoi/report/lunds/3_3.htm*).

3 This is based on information from Rengo (Japanese Trade Union Confederation) (2005), Let's Start Action 2005; Spring Struggle for a Better Life (Rengo's policies for the 2005 Spring Struggle (*Syunki Seikatsu Tosō*).

4 Despite the aim to coordinate, home help is still regulated by the Law for Social Services of 1991, while home nursing is still regulated by the law passed in 1984 concerning municipal health. Thus no unified law was passed during this development.

Chapter 3

1 There were some charity works for poor elderly in Japan even before 1962. Sasaki shows an example of charity work by a lady past middle age in the Municipality of Ueda, Nagano Prefecture. The lady visited elderly

to talk with them, and she also visited widows to help. The lady was a Christian and had three grown-up children, and she helped such people because she could not ignore them (Sasaki 2005: 78).

2 There are examples of home help in some municipalities before 1962. For example, Nagano Prefecture contracted out home help services ('Dispatching of home helpers in Nagano Prefecture' (*Nagano-ken Katei Yōgofu Haken Jigyō*)) to six municipalities, five towns, and twelve villages in 1956. Some researchers argue that Nagano was the first example of home help services in Japan. The Municipality of Osaka introduced temporary dispatching of home helpers in 1959 for elderly who lived alone and needed social assistance. Services included laundry, cleaning, sewing, and other kinds of care. Widows and single mothers in need of social assistance were often employed as home helpers. The municipalities of Kobe, Nagoya, and Tokyo also introduced 'Dispatching of home helpers' before the government introduced this service in 1962 (Takaki 2006: 20; Kitaba 2001: 209; Sasaki 2005: 77–81; Suga 2001: 47–8).

3 Home helpers were called 'home servants for the elderly' (*rōjin katei hōshiin*) at that time. Bureaucrats in the Ministry of Health and Welfare were aware of the English words 'home helper' and 'home maker,' but thought that English names were not suitable for the Japanese public administrative system (Mori 1974: 7). From 1989, however, 'home helper' (*hōmu herupa-*) was used, even in official documents; since 2000 'visiting careworker' (*hōmon kaigoin*) has been officially used.

4 Social welfare corporations (*Shakai fukushi hōjin*). A corporate status provided for under Articles 5 and 22 of the Social Welfare Services Law (*Shakai fukushi jigyō hō*), whereby a private welfare administrative organization can be accredited to provide specified publicly recognized welfare services and receive public financing for these programs (Nakamura, Kojima, and Thompson 1981: 13–14).

5 [Translator's note]: the Imperial Rescript on Education, signed by Emperor Meiji in 1890, articulated the Meiji government's educational principles. Students were required to memorize the full text. It stressed, among other things, filial piety as the fundamental relationship between children and parents, and that a parent/child relationship should exist based on loyalty between imperial subjects and the Emperor.

6 Management outline of home helpers (*Rōjin Katei Hōshiinn jigyō unei yōkō*) was revised by the Ministry of Health and Welfare in 1982.

7 The Alzheimer's Association of Japan is a non-profit nationwide organization concerned with people with dementia (including Alzheimer's disease)

and their family caregivers. Purposes of the organization are to promote policies for people with dementia and their families. The first demand for better support for families bearing the burden of care was made to the Minister of Health and Welfare in 1982, which handled dementia issues. The association has forty-one local offices, which means that almost every prefecture has a local office, as there are forty-seven prefectures in Japan. The local offices are very active in helping people with dementia and their families. For example, they offer telephone advice services for families who take care of people with dementia, and they research and make suggestions for better care for people with dementia. When first established, the Japanese name was *Boke rōjin wo kakaeru kazoku no kai* but this was later changed to *Ninchishō no hito to kazoku no kai* (http://www2f.biglobe.ne.jp [July 10, 2009]).

8 The Women's Association for the Better Aging Society was established in March 1983 following the 'Women's Symposium on the Problems of Aging' in September 1982. There are 1200 members and eighty-seven member groups from all over the country. Members include scholars, researchers, medical specialists, welfare workers, journalists, and wives who have the burden of caring for aged persons. The Japanese name is *Kourei shakai wo yokusuru jyosei no kai*. The society's activities include surveying the problems of an aged society from the viewpoint of women, as well as issuing warnings and offering suggestions (addressed to both the general public and the government) concerning the problems of an aged society (http://www7.ocn.ne.jp [July 10, 2009]).

9 Ministry of Health and Welfare (1938–2000). Reorganization of government ministries and agencies resulted in consolidation with the Ministry of Labour, leading to the creation of the Ministry of Health, Labour, and Welfare in 2001.

10 The municipal elderly care plans (*Rōjin Hoken Fukushi Keikaku*), under the Law for the Welfare of the Elderly in 1990, obligated all municipalities to make their own elderly care plans. The first municipal elderly care plans were published in 1994. In the beginning, municipal plans had to be made every five years, but every three years since 2000.

11 See note 4.

12 In the 1993 election, the Liberal Democratic Party (LDP) did not get a majority in the House of Representatives. Non-LDP coalition governments were the Hosokawa coalition government (July 1993–April 1994) and the Hata coalition government (April–June 1994). The LDP created a coalition with the Social Democratic Party (SDP) and the New Party SAKIGAKE (NPS) to return to government in June 1994. This

was the Murayama coalition government (June 1994–August 1995), with SDP leader Tomiichi Murayama acting as Prime Minister. The LDP, the SDP, and the NPS coalition government continued until the Hashimoto coalition government (August 1995–July 1998) came to power in a new mixed of coalition partners.

13 'The research committee of elderly care and self-independence' (*Koureisya kaigo jiritsu shien shisutemu kenkyūkai*) was a research group that consisted of researchers, medical specialists, and bureaucrats in the Ministry of Health and Welfare and held some research meetings in 1994. The idea of the LTCI System came from its report.

14 The Japanese Trade Union Confederation (Rengo, 6.8 million members (2007)). Japanese trade union organizations have a three-tier hierarchical structure: enterprise-based unions, industrial federations, and the national center at the top. There is also a wide-ranging network with local organizations, called 'Local Rengos,' set up in all of Japan's prefectures (*http://www.jtuc-rengo.org/about/index.html* [July 10, 2009]).

15 In-home services (*kyotaku sa-bisu*) include home help services, home visit bathing service, home visit nursing, home visit rehabilitation, management guidance for in-home care, rental service of welfare equipment, and day service.

16 See note 4.

17 The National Council of Social Welfare (*Zenkoku shakai fukushi kyōgi kai*) was incorporated as a social welfare corporation (*Shakai fukushi hōjin*) in 1951. The purpose is to promote and organize activities of non-governmental social welfare agencies, and to develop the efficient administration of social welfare throughout the country. Now all prefectures and municipalities must have a council of social welfare as per the Social Welfare Law (*Shakai fukushi hō*) (Article 109). The Social Welfare Service Law (*Shakai fukushi jigyō hō*) changed to the Social Welfare Law in 2000.

18 COMSN was the biggest private care provider in Japan before the incident (see Chapter 7).

19 The questionnaire changed as from April 2009. The previous number of eighty-four questions has been reduced to seventy-four. According to the Ministry of Health, Labour, and Welfare, the number of frail elderly who are assessed as 'independent' almost doubled in April–May 2009 compared with the number in April–May 2008 (Mainichi, and Sankei Newspaper, July 13, 2009). People assessed as being in the 'independent' level cannot be given any benefit. It means that the new questionnaire works to reduce benefits.

20 People who are over sixty-five pay the LTCI premium. The premium depends on their income and municipality. A standard premium was 4160 yen (U.S. dollar (US$) 45.65/Euro (EUR) 30.53) per month in 2009. The standard premium has increased from 2911 yen (US$31.94/EUR21.35) in 2000, 3293 yen (US$36.14/EUR21.46) in 2003, and 4090 yen (US$44.88/EUR30.01) in 2006.
21 'Housework support' (*kaji enjyo*) changed its name to 'daily life support' (*seikatsu shien*) in 2003.
22 Notification from the manager of Policy Promotion, Division of Health and Welfare of Elderly, No. 76 (*Roujin-hoken-fukushi-kyoku shinkō-ka katyō tsuuchi dai 76 gō*).

Chapter 4

1 This chapter was based on "Long-Term Care Insurance, marketization and the quality of care: 'Good time living' in a recently established nursing home in a suburb of Tokyo," by Reiko Abe Auestad (2009), *Japan Forum* vol.21(2), Journal of the British Association for Japanese Studies. I would like to thank the anonymous readers and the editor of *Japan Forum* for their insightful critical comments. Thanks are also due to Yayoi Saitō, Anne Thelle, and Karen Christensen for their guidance and assistance.
2 For a discussion of the historical background for the emergence of the *Japanese-style welfare society*, see Goodman 2002: 15.
3 The insurance fees are paid by those over the age of sixty-five, the *primary insured*, and those between forty and sixty-four, the *secondary insured*. The secondary insured are allowed to apply for services only when they are suffering from special illnesses such as Alzheimer's and Parkinson's disease.
4 See Ainoya, Kakiuchi, and Ogawa 2001, Katō 2001, and Sakamoto 2003, for example.
5 The upper limit of the 10% charge for non-low income persons is 37,200 yen/month, while for old-age welfare pension recipients it is 15,000 yen/month. See http://www.mhlw.go.jp/english/topics/elderly/care/index.html.
6 The number of homes has increased from 350 in 2000 to 1045 in 2004, an increase of 50.6% compared to 2003 (Morimiya 2006: 101).
7 In contrast to their United States counterparts, licensed private senior housing in Japan is required to meet the Japanese government's specification as to unit size and services offered (Osako 2006: 1).

8 Katsuko Morimiya writes that prior to the introduction of the LTCI, it was common for private nursing homes to charge thirty to fifty million yen as an initial deposit besides the monthly fees, whereas now we find many private nursing homes with an initial deposit of around five million yen or even lower (Morimiya 2006: 101). For other statistical data on private nursing homes, see Morimiya's essay, and also Yuki 2008: 43.

9 According to the 2002 survey by the Ministry of Health, Labour, and Welfare, the majority of families with heavily dependent elderly did not use the maximum allocated amount of the LTCI and the biggest reason for this was 'because they managed to get by with help from their families' (Nakai 2004: 60). This demonstrates that there are still many households, regardless of their incomes, that would prefer to rely on their families (often daughters and daughters-in-law) than to have to pay for the LTCI.

10 Kittay (1999: 9–17) gives a review of feminist critiques of equality by dividing them into three variants: the difference critique, the diversity critique, and the dependency critique, the last of which forms the basis of her thesis.

11 For discussions that problematize the traditional model of the care of the elderly that relies heavily on family (daughters-in-law and daughters) and call for socialization of care, see Sugimoto 1997, Kasuga 2001, and Banzai 1999, for example.

12 Using the notion of *emotional labor* developed by Russell Arlie Hochschild, Kisuyo Kasuga discusses the need for cultivating a new, more expansive notion of care that goes beyond mechanical, physical assistance. She warns, however, against the danger that the focus on the emotional aspect of care labor can strengthen the conventional and essentialist view of women as the most suitable caregivers (Kasuga 2003: 235). See also Kasaya 2004.

13 Yayoi Saito (2008) describes the social orientation as marketable profile in many of the care providers independently of their status as organizations. Interestingly, she points out that there are for-profit agencies with a strong social and community-oriented profile, while there are profit-oriented social welfare foundations.

14 The other Gasshōsen facilities include Homes for the Elderly (*yōgo rōjin hōmu*) and Special Nursing Homes (*Tokubetsu yōgo rōjin hōmu*, often abbreviated as *tokuyō*).

15 The old *ie* ideal of the hierarchical and yet synergic intergenerational relationship bound by an exchange of care and inheritance remains strong in many parts of Japan, even though many have realized it has become a rather unrealistic ideal. Judging from the critics' description of the *ie* mentality surviving in contemporary Japan, we have reason to believe

Table N.1 Monthly expenses in Tsuru no sato (2008)

Admission fee	7,980,000 yen
Monthly expenses	
Monthly rent	120,000 yen
Meals (three times a day)	57,750 yen
Facility fees	68,250 yen
Total monthly expenses	246,000 yen

that the image of the thrifty elderly parents who scrape and save every penny to pass on their inheritance in exchange for the care and attention from their children's family (usually women) still lives on. See Sugimoto 1997, Kasuga 2001, and Banzai 1999.

16 The accounts of the living condition and the residents' lives in Tsuru no sato are based on my observations made during my stay as an in-house guest in July and November 2007. The details of the cost of living at Tsuru no sato (Tsuru no sato 2008) are outlined in Table N.1. The expenses for senior apartments are the initial fee of about 100 million yen plus monthly rent/management of about 100,000 yen for an apartment of between fifty to fifty-five square meters. See *http://www.gsen.or.jp/tsurunosato*.

17 One week's menu in November 2007: clam chowder, sautéed sausages and cabbage, and salad; mackerel cooked in miso-based sauce in a Japanese way; Chinese chop-suy with vegetables and pork; sautéed chicken and eggplant with Chinese sauce; thinly sliced beef stewed in tomato sauce; hamburger with grated radish; rolled cabbage Japanese style; grilled eel Japanese style at an extra cost of 400 yen; deep-fried scallops at an extra cost of 400 yen; sashimi at an extra cost of 400 yen.

18 In Tsuru no sato, one-third of the residents are categorized as either independent or at dependency level 1 or 2. The general level of disability among residents in an equivalent Norwegian nursing homes would be presumably much higher.

19 Of the sixty-seven residents in Tsuru no sato, forty-seven are women and the average age is 86.1 as of September 2, 2008.

20 See, for example, the homepages for private homes run by Watami, Alive, and Best life: *http://www.wataminokaigo.net/feature/index.html*, *http://www.alive-carehome.co.jp/about/voice_profile.html*, and *http://www.bestlife.jp/aboutus/living.html*.

21 See *http://www.wataminokaigo.net/care/food.html*, and *http://www.alive-carehome.co.jp/about/indicate_oneday-s2.html* and the homepage for Nichii, *http://www.nichii-home.jp/home/tama.html.*

22 A focus on its hotel-like regime with key concepts such as *guests first* and *good time living*, which inspired Tsuru no sato, naturally seems to be a common feature of the senior housing projects run by Mitsuru Haruyama's Orix Corp. See *http://www.orixliving.jp/goodtimeliving/about/concept.html.*

23 This is called the LEON principle (a Norwegian abbreviation for *lowest effective care level*), and emphasizes the cost-effective use of resources in home help services (Larsen 2008). See also *http://www.forebygging.no/fhp/d_emneside/cf/hPKey_808/hParent_8/hDKey_1.*

24 As far as nursing homes are concerned, one might say it is more correct to say 'equal inaccessibility.'

25 My accounts of Norwegian nursing homes are based on my visits to two municipal nursing homes and one private nursing home in the Oslo region in September 2008. Nesoddtunet bo- og servicesenter in Nesodden, just outside Oslo (public), Kantarellen bo- og rehabiliteringssenter in Oslo (public), and St Halvardshjemmet (private).

26 This observation was made at Kantalleren bo- og servicesenter. It should be noted, however, that private nursing homes such as St Halvardshjemmet run by a Christian organization, Kirkens bymisjon, emphasize the importance of organized weekly, if not daily, cultural activities for their residents. They also try to create their own distinct profile according to their Christian values.

27 A resident at the Kantalleren bo- og servicesenter.

28 A remark made by a care worker at Kantalleren bo- og servicesenter.

29 Mr D., who immigrated to Oslo in the 1960s.

30 Practical assistance (as opposed to the home-nursing assistance) in the home-help services in Oslo was partly privatized in 2006, and 20% of the users now choose private providers rather than those run by municipalities. Many private providers advertise their readiness to send the same person to one client to avoid fragmentation of the care work. The privatization process in nursing homes is slowly underway in municipalities with large populations, even though it does not seem to have helped the waiting list problem. Twenty-two of the fifty-one nursing homes in Oslo, four of the sixteen in Stavanger, and four of the twenty-four in Trondheim are run by private organizations.

31 The place of residence is a neglected factor under the LTCI System in Japan because the forces of privatization have naturally had most impact

in big cities with large populations. Out of 648 private nursing homes in Japan, as many as 508 are in Tokyo, Kanagawa, and Saitama. Comparing the nursing home situation in scarcely populated areas in Japan and in Norway may be a worthwhile project, even though it is beyond the scope of the present paper.

32 The legally supported mutual dependence system behind the *ie* ideology was dismantled when the 1947 constitution abolished it by giving all the siblings an equal right to inherit (the eldest son who takes care of the parents was no longer the head of of the *ie*). The *ie* mentality has, however, lingered on, and many eldest sons and their wives have felt obliged to live up to the expectations of the previous generation without the compensation in material and symbolic values they used to have.

33 She continues: the biggest change after the introduction of the care insurance system is the subversion of the commonsense view that 'the old [are] best cared for in the hands of the family' in a very short period of time (Ueno 2007:178).

34 The 2006 revision in the Nursing Care Insurance Law addresses a number of pressing issues, one of which is emphasizing the preventive care for the elderly that can promote their self-sufficiency (*Japan Times* 2005).

Chapter 5

1 I use the words *recipient* and *user* interchangeably to denote the person who receives home help through the social and health care system.

2 Several senior social welfare researchers have underscored this dualism of care work; see, for example, Thorsen (2003), where she argues that the purpose of home help services is to give services with care—care being conceptualized holistically as relation-focused help. According to Wærness, the care-giving work contains a practical side as well as an emotional side (Wærness 1982, 1999). Szebehely has pointed out that care work is performed within personal relation ties between caregiver and care recipient, and that an instrumental attitude to care work is irreconcilable with good care giving (Szebehely 1995).

3 Also individual characteristics of the care worker such as own moral standards, values, and attitudes have an impact on the extent to which relational power will be exerted. Moreover, care workers vary in their ability to empathize and with regard to their experiences and qualifications. However, these are not addressed in this study.

4 The data was collected as part of the author's doctoral study at the Norwegian University of Science and Technology in Norway. The data collection was to a great extent financed by a grant from the Univers Foundation, which the author gratefully acknowledges.

5 In Japan data was collected prior to the implementation of the revision of the LTCI System in April 2006.

6 According to an independent samples test, this is significant (level of Sig. 05) for concluding that, in general, home helpers in Japan are a few years (around three years) older than in Norway. Test results are not presented in this report, but most of the findings reported here are significant, i.e. we can with a high degree of probability conclude that the differences between the samples in the survey also hold true for the population of home helpers in the two countries.

7 For instance, in Japan certain helpers do bodily care (*shintai kaigo*), while others do housework (*seikatsu enjo*), and some do both, depending among other things on their qualifications (Level 1, 2, or 3), and what they, themselves, prefer to do. In Norway help with bodily care such as bathing is normally designated to visiting nurses, not to home helpers.

8 As for cleaning, one municipality in Norway has established a larger center covering the whole city and specializing in home help services only in terms of cleaning. Home helpers in this municipality work in teams of two helpers, which means that they have twice as many recipients to visit compared to working alone. On a normal work day they clean in the homes of as many as eleven recipients, which also increases the time spent on travel. Needless to say, this is very stressful and hard.

9 The questionnaire had one question asking the helpers if any of the recipients they go to regularly is demented. Ninety percent of the Norwegian helpers said yes, compared to 70% in Japan. As for the question whether any of their recipients ought to be in a nursing home, 52% of Japanese home helpers think so, compared to three-quarters of the Norwegian helpers, indicating just how dependent many recipients are on help and the need for additional time in many instances.

10 I would like to emphasize that this is based on data that was collected prior to the implementation of the revision of the LTCI System in April 2006.

11 The figure from Norway is the basic salary from the wage list for public employees, while the figure from Japan is based on interview data.

Chapter 8

1 NEET (young people Not in Education, Employment, or Training) was first used in the United Kingdom. According to the Ministry of Health, Labor, and Welfare in Japan, the growth in the NEET population was estimated at 520,000 in September 2003.

2 *Hikikomori* (social withdrawal) is a Japanese term to refer to the phenomenon of reclusive individuals who have chosen to withdraw from social life. The term refers to both the sociological phenomenon in general, as well as to individuals belonging to this societal group.

3 *Sotokomori* is a Japanese term to refer to the phenomenon of people who live in other countries where people can live more cheaply than in Japan, after they earn money in a certain period.

4 SOHO (Small Office Home Office) is a kind of working style in which people work at home with computers, telephones, and the internet.

Bibliography

Introduction

Kuhnle, Stein 1990. Den skandinaviske velferdsmodellen-skandinavisk? velferd? modell? (The Scandinavian welfare model-scandinavian? welfare? model?), i Anders Rosenhayn Hovdum, Stein Kuhnle and Liv Stokke, (red.), *Visjoner om velferdssamfunnet* (Vision of the welfare society), Alma Mater, Bergen.

Petersson, Olof 2000. *Nordisk politik, femte upplagan* (Politics in the Nordic countries. The fifth edition), Norstedts juridik: Stockholm.

Tsubogō, Minoru 2007. 'Fukushi tagen shugi no jidai' (Pluralism in the welfare society) in Norio Okazawa (eds.), *Fukushi governansu sengen* (Social welfare governance in Japan) Nihon keizai hyōron sha), p. 228.

Chapter 1

Abrahamsson, Bengt and Mårten Söder (1977), *Makten och verksamheten. Om villkor och verksamhet vid vårdhemsavdelingar*, Uppsala: Acta Universitas Upsaliensis.

Abrams, P. (1977), 'Community care: some research problems and priorities', *Policy and Politics,* 6 (2), pp. 125–51.

Alvsvag, Herdis (1981), *Har sykepleien en fremtid?*, Oslo: Universitetsforlaget.

Bell, D. (1968), 'The measurement of knowledge and technology,' in E. B. Sheldon and W. E. Moore (eds.), *Indicators of Social Change*, New York: Russell Sage Foundation.

Bernstein, Basil (1975), *Class, Codes and Control*, New York: Schocken.

Branca, Patricia (1975), *Silent Sisterhood: Middle-class Women in the Victorian Home*, Croom Helm.

Daatland, Sven Olav (1983), 'Eldrecomsorgeni en småby de offentlige hjelpetjenester og familiens rolle' (Elderly care in a small village: the public home care services and the role of the family), in *Tidsskrift för samfunnsforskning*, 2, pp. 155–73.

Dawe, Alan (1978), 'Theories of social action,' in T. Bottomore and Robert Nisbet (eds.), *A History of Sociological Analysis,* New York: Basic Books.
de Beauvoir, Simone (1953), *The Second Sex*, New York: Bantam Books.
Donzelot, Jacques (1979), *The Policing of Families*, Hutchinson.
Ehrenreich, Barbara and Deidre English (1973), *Witches, Midwives and Nurses: A History of Women Healers*, New York: Feminist Press.
Finch, Janet and Dulcie Groves (1980), 'Community care and the family: a case for equal opportunities?', *Journal of Social Policy*, 9 (4), pp. 487–511.
Firestone, Shulamit (1971), *The Dialectics of Sex*, New York: Bantam Books.
Freidson, Eliot (1973), 'Professions and their occupational principle,' in E. Freidson (ed.), *The Professions and their Prospects*, Beverly Hills: Sage.
Friedan, Betty (1963), *The Feminine Mystique*, New York: Dell.
Friedan, Betty (1981), *The Second Stage*, New York: Summit Books.
Glennon, Lynda M. (1979), *Women and Dualism: A Sociology of Knowledge Analysis*, New York: Longman.
Gullestad, Marianne (1984), *Kitchen-table Society: A Case Study of the Family Life and Friendship of Young Working Class Women in Urban Norway*, Oslo: Universitetsforlaget.
Hochschild, Arlie Russell (1975), 'The sociology of feelings and emotion: selected possibilities,' in M. Millman and R. M. Kanter (eds.), *Another Voice*, New York: Anchor Books.
Holter, Harriet, Willy Martinussen, and Bjørg Grønseth (1967), *Hjemmet som arbeidsplass. Studier av husmorens arbeids—situasjon, av veiledningsbehov og veiledningtilbud* (Home as a working place: studies of the work situation of housewives, their needs and supply of information), Oslo: Universitets forlaget.
Illich, Ivan (1976), *Medical Nemesis*, New York: Random House.
Kitzinger, Sheila (1978), *Women as Mothers*, Fontana.
Levin, Lowell S. and Ellen S. Idler (1981), *The Hidden Health Care System: Mediating Structures and Medicine*, Cambridge, MA: Harper and Row.
Liljeström, Rita and Elizabeth Özgalda (1980), *Kommunals kvinnor på livets trappa* (Women workers of the Swedish municipal workers union on the stairs of life), Stockholm: Svenska kommunalarbetareförbundet.
List, Elizabeth (1983), 'The science of the fathers and the science of the sons: reflection on a feminist critique of science' (working paper), Graz: Institut of für philosophie.
Lopata, Helena Znaniecki (1971), *Occupation: Housewife*, Oxford University Press.

Martinsen, Kari and Kari Wærness (1979), *Pleie uten omsorg?* (Nursing without care?), Oslo: Pax Forlag.

McMillan, Carol (1982), *Women, Reason and Nature: Some Philosophical Problems with Feminism*, Oxford: Basil Blackwell.

Merton, Robert K. and Elinor Barber (1967), 'Sociological ambivalence,' in E. A. Tiryakian (ed.), *Sociological Theory, Values and Sociocultural Change*, New York: Harper Torchbooks.

Millett, Kate (1971), *Sexual Politics*, New York: Avon Books.

Mitchell, Juliet (1971), *Women's Estate*, Penguin.

Moroney, R. M. (1976), *The Family and State Considerations for Social Policy*, Longman.

Newson, John and Elizabeth (1976), *Patterns of Infant Care in an Urban Community*, Pelican.

Nordhus, Inger Hilde (1981), *Gammel og avhengig?* (Old and dependent?), Bergen: Department of Psychology, University of Bergen.

O'Brien, Mary (1981), *The Politics of Reproduction*, Routledge and Kegan Paul.

Oakley, Ann (1974), *The Sociology of Housework*, New York: Pantheon Books.

Oakley, Ann (1976), 'Wisewoman and medicine man: changes in the management of childbirth,' in Juliet Mitchell and Ann Oakley (eds.), *The Rights and Wrongs of Women*, Penguin.

Pensionärundersökningens rapporter om social hemhjälp m.m. (1979), Stockholm: Socialdepartmentet Ds S: 5.

'Psychosocial conditions for development in early childhood' (1973), Fifth International Seminar on Health Education, Schmallenberg, 25–29 June, *International Journal of Health Education*.

Ressner, Ulla (1981), *Vårdarbetar* kollektivet *och facket* (The care workers' collective and the labor union), Stockholm: The Swedish Centre for Working Life.

Rosenmayr, L. and E. Köckeis (1965), 'Propositions for a sociology of aging and the family,' in R. Winch and L. Goodman (eds.), *Selected Studies in Marriage and the Family*, New York.

Schaffer, Rudolf (1977), *Mothering*, Fontana.

Schorr, Alvan (1962), 'Current practice of filial responsibility' in R. Winch R. McGunnis and H. Barringer (eds.), *Selected Studies in Marriage and the Family*, New York.

Schumacher, E. F. (1978), *A Guide for the Perplexed*, Abacus, Sphere Books.

Sennett, Richard and Jonathan Cobb (1972), *The Hidden Injuries of Class*, New York: Knopf.

Shanas, Ethel (1979), 'Social myth as hypothesis: the case of the family relations of old people,' *The Gerontologist,* 19 (1), pp. 3–9.

Smith, Dorothy I. (1979), 'A sociology for women,' in J. A. Sherman and E. J. Beck (eds.), *The Prism of Sex*, Madison: University of Wisconsin Press.

Stacey, Margaret (1981), 'The division of labour revisited or overcoming the two Adams,' in Philip Abrams et al. (eds.), *Practice and Progress: British Sociology 1950–1980*, Allen & Unwin, pp. 174–5.

Stacey, Margaret and Marion Price (1981), *Women, Power and Politics*, Tavistock Publications Ltd.

Sundström, Gerdt (1982), 'The elderly, women's work and social security costs,' *Acta Sociologica,* 25 (1).

Söder, Mårten (1981), *Vårdintegration, vårdideologi och integrering* (Integration of care services, care ideology, and integration of care receivers), Uppsala: Acta Universitas Upsaliensis, Abstracts of Uppsala Dissertations from the Faculty of Social Sciences, 25.

Teeland, Lawrence (1978) *Keeping in touch*, Monograph 16 Gothenberg: Department of Sociology, University of Gothenberg.

Titmuss, Richard M. (1963), *Essays on the Welfare State*, Boston: Beacon Press.

Ve, Hildur (1982), 'Ideals of equality in the school system of the welfare state,' paper presented at the Tenth World Congress of Sociology, Research Group 32: *Women in Society*, Mexico, 16–21 August, Bergen: Center of Women's Studies, Institute of Sociology.

Viklund, Rune (1981), *Att arbela i omsorg* (Working in care services), Stockholm: The Center for Working Life.

Weber, Max (1966), *The Theory of Social and Economic Organization*, New York: The Free Press.

Webster's New World Dictionary of the American Language (1976), Cleveland, Ohio: World Publishing Company.

Wærness, Kari (1978), 'The invisible welfare state: women's work at home,' in *Acta Sociologica* Supplement.

Wærness, Kari (1982), *Kvinneperspektiver på sosialpolitikken* (Social policy from women's perspectives), Oslo: Universitetsforlaget.

Chapter 2

Abrams, Philip (1982), *Historical Sociology*, Ithaca, NY: Cornell University Press.

Askheim, Ole Petter (2003), *Fra normalisering til empowerment. Ideologier og praksis i arbeid med funksjonshemmede* (From normalisation to empowerment. Ideologies and praxis of working with disabled people.), Oslo: Gyldendal Norsk Forlag.

Auestad, Reiko Abe (2005), 'Familie og kvinner i japansk populærkultur: Kjønsroller i endring eller i tilpasning?' (Family and women in Japanese popular culture. Changing of adapting gender roles?) in Grønning, T. (ed.): Vinduer mot Japan (Windows towards Japan). Tapir akademisk forlag.

Bauman, Zygmunt (2005), *Work, Consumerism and the New Poor*, Maidenhead: Open University Press.

Bogen, Hanne (2001), 'Hvilke konsekvenser har konkurranseutsetting for ansatte?' (What are the consequences of outsourcing for employees?) in *Tidsskrift for Velferdsforskning* (Journal of Welfare Research), vol.4, no.4, pp.207–21.

Bogen, H. and Nyen, T. (1998), *Privatisering og konkurranseutsetting i norske kommuner* (Privatization and outsourcing in Norwegian municipalities), Fafo-report 254, Oslo: Fafo (Institute for Applied Social Science).

Bungum, Brita (1994), *Effektivisering av omsorg. Kjønnsperspektiv på omstilling av offentlig omsorgsarbeid* (Increasing the efficient of care. Gender perspective on reorganization of public care work.) Report from LOS-project 'Mulighetsstrukttturer i offentlige og private foretak,' (Option structures in public and private enterprises) University of Trondheim: Institute of Sociology and Political Science.

Christensen, Karen (1998a), 'Andre-orientering og omsorgsarbejde' (Other orientation and care work) in *Tidsskrift for Velferdsforskning* (Journal of Welfare Research), vol.1, no.2, pp. 82–96.

Christensen, Karen (1998b), *Omsorg og arbejde. En sociologisk studie af ændringer i den hjemmebaserede omsorg* (Care and work. A sociological study of changes in home based care). Dissertation. University of Bergen: Department of Sociology.

Christensen, Karen (2001), 'Mellem politikken og folket. De sociale tjenesters græsrodsbureaukrater og deres fordelingspraksis (Between politics and people. The street level bureaucrats of social services, and their praxis of distribution),' in *Tidsskrift for velferdsforskning* (Journal of Welfare Research), vol. 4, no.4, pp. 222–38.

Christensen, Karen (2005), The modernization of power in Norwegian home care services,' in H. M. Dahl and T. Rask Eriksen (eds.), Dilemmas of Care in the Nordic Welfare State: Continuity and Change, Aldershot: Ashgate, pp.33-46.

Christensen, Karen and Sturle Næss (1999), *Kunnskapsstatus om de offentlige omsorgstjenestene* (Knowledge status about the public care services),

Bergen: Senter for samfunnsforskning (SEFOS) (Center for social research).

Edvardsen, Unni (2005): 'Omsorgsutfordringer i et aldrende Japan,' (Care challenges in an ageing Japan) in Grønning, T. (ed.): Vinduer mot Japan (Windows towards Japan). Tapir akademisk forlag.

Eliasson, Rosmari (1987), *Forskningsetik og perspektivval* (Research ethics and choice of perspective), FoU-reportt 7A, Stockholms socialförvaltning, Stockholm: Forsknings- och utvecklingsbyrån (Research and development office).

Eliasson, Rosmari (1992), 'Omsorg som lönarbete: om taylorisering och professionalisering,' (Care and paid work: on taylorization and professionalization) pp.131–42 in Eliasson (red.), *Egenheter och allmänheter.* En antologi om omsorg och omsorgens villkor (Peculiarities and generalities: An antology about care care conditions), Lund: Arkiv förlag.

Esping-Andersen, Gøsta (1990), *The Three Worlds of Welfare Capitalism*, Cambridge: Polity Press.

Esping-Andersen, Gøsta (1999), *Social Foundations of Postindustrial Economies*, Oxford: University Press.

Giddens, Anthony (1982), *Sociology: A Brief but Critical Introduction*, San Diego, CA: Harcourt Brace Jovanovich.

Høst, Håkon (1997), *Konstruksjonen av omsorgsarbeideren* (The construction of the care worker), AHS serie 2/97, Bergen: Arbeidsliv-Historie-Samfunn, Gruppe for flerfaglig arbeidsforskning (Working life-history-society. Group for cross disciplinary research on work)

Lie, Bente (1987), *Et yrke tar form. En analyse av hjemmehjelpernes yrkesrolle og yrkesdanning* (An occupation takes shape. An analysis of the occupation role and occupation education of home helpers), Master thesis, University of Oslo: Department of sociology..

Næss, Sturle and Kari Wærness (1996), *Bedre omsorg? Kommunal eldreomsorg 1980–95* (Better care? Municipal elderly care 1980-95), Bergen: Senter for samfunnsforskning (SEFOS) (Center for social research).

Nielsen, Rune Åkvik (2007), 'Før var alt fast, nå er alt flytende: En kritikk av Zygmunt Baumans samtidsdiagnose' (Earlier everything was regular, now everything is liquid: Critisizing Zygmunt Bauman's diagnosis of present time) in *Sosiologisk tidsskrift* (Journal of Sociology), 15 (1), pp. 3–27.

NOU (Norges offentlige utredning) (Norwegian public report) (1986), 4 *Samordning i helse- og sosialtjenesten* (Coordination of health- and social services), Oslo: Universitetsforlaget.

Ones, Torunn (1988), *Organisering av omsorgsarbeid* (Organizing care work), Master thesis in health- and social policy, University of Bergen.

Pedersen, Anne Reff (2001), 'Fortællinger om hjemmeplejens organisering' (Narratives about the organization of home nursing services) pp.84–112 in Skånning Nielsen og Lomborg (red.), *På arbejde i hjemmet* (Working at home), København: Gyldendal.

Rønning, Rolf (1995), 'Kvalitet i hjemmehjelpstjenestene – en lokal studie (Quality in home help services – a local study),' i *Aldring og Eldre* (Ageing and older people), 1, pp.2–7, Oslo: Universitetsforlaget.

Saito, Yayoi (2002), 'Elderly care policy in Japan during the 20th century: historic review and prospect for the 21st century,' in *Challenges for Japan –Democracy, Busines and Aging–*, pp. 191–217, International House of Japan.

St. meld. nr. 25 (2005-06), *Mestring, muligheter og mening. Framtidas omsorgsutfordringer.* (Report to the Storting: Mastering, possibilities and meaning. Care challenges of the future), Helse- og omsorgesdepartementet (The Norwegian Health Care Department).

Szebehely, Marta (1995), *Vardagens organisering. Om vårdbiträden och gamla i Hemtjänsten* (Organizing everyday life. On home helpers and old people in home help services), Stockholm: Arkiv.

Taylor, Frederick Winslow (1916), *The Principles of Scientific Management*, New York: Harper & Brothers.

Tönnies, Ferdinand (1963), *Community and Society:* (Gemeinschaft und Gesellschaft), translated and edited by Charles P. Loomis, New York : Harper & Row.

Vabø, Mia (2001), '(For)brukerorientering og omsorg' (Consumer orientation and care) in Thorsen, Dahle og Vabø *Makt og avmakt i helse- og omsorgstjenestene* (Power and powerlessness in health- and care services), Oslo: NOVA-report 18/2001.Norsk institutt for forskning om oppvekst, velferd og aldring. (Norwegian institute for research into childhood, welfare and ageing).

Wærness, Kari (1982), *Kvinneperspektiver på sosialpolitikken* (Women perspectives on social politics), Oslo, Bergen, Tromsø: Universitetsforlaget.

Wærness, Kari (1984), 'The rationality of caring,' in *Economic and Industrial Democracy*, 5, pp. 185–211.

Wærness, Kari (1996), 'Omsorgsrationalitet. Reflexioner över et begrepps karriär' (Care rationality. Reflections about the career of a concept), pp. 203–20 in Eliasson (red.), *Omsorgens skiftninger* (The changes of care), Lund: Studentlitteratur.

Weber, Max (1994), *Makt og byråkrati* (Power and bureaucracy), Oslo: Gyldendal Norsk Forlag.

Chapter 3

Akeyama, Kazuo and T. Nogawa (1975), 'Rōjin katei hōshiin seido—enkaku, genjō, tenbō' (The home servants for elderly homes system—history, actual conditions, prospects), in Ōta Takeo (ed.), *Gendai no oyako mondai* (Contemporary parent–child problems), Tokyo: Yūhikaku. pp. 324–349.

Arai, Yasutomo (2004), Ho-muherupu rōdō no henshitsu ni tsuite—ho-muherupu seisaku no shiten kara—ho-muherupu seisaku no shiten kara (The transformation in home help work; from the viewpoint of home-help policy), *Hagoromo Gakuen Tankidaigaku kenkyū kihyō*, vol. 40. pp. 1–9.

Christensen, Karen (2004), 'The modernization of power in Norwegian home care services,' in Hanne Marlene Dahl and Tine Rask Eriksen (eds), *Dilemmas of Care in the Nordic Welfare State: Continuity and Change*, Ashgate. pp. 33–46.

Christensen, Karen (2005), 'Social capital in public home care services (1)', in Sirpa Wrede, Lea Henriksson, Håkon Høst, Stina Johansson and Betina Dybbroe (eds), *Care Work in Crisis: Reclaiming the Nordic Ethos of Care*, Malmö, Sweden: Studentlitteratur, pp. 249–71.

Goodman, Roger and Peng Ito (1996), 'The East Asian welfare state: peripatetic learning, adaptive changes and nation-building,' in Gøsta Esping-Andersen (ed.), *Welfare States in Transition: National Adaptations in Global Economies*, London: Sage Publications. pp. 192–224.

Kitaba, Tsutomu (2001), 'Waga kuni ni okeru zaitaku fukushi seisaku no tenkai katei—rōjin hōshiin hakken seido no kaihatsu wo chūshin ni' (The development process of policy concerning in-home care in Japan: with a focus on the evolution of the dispatch system of home servants for the elderly), *Nihon Shakaikigyō daigaku kenkyū kihyō*, vol. 48. pp. 207–242.

Mori, Mikio (1974), *Ho-muherupu* (Home helpers), *Zaidanhojin nihon seimei saiseikai syakai jimukyoku.*

Nakamura Yūichi, Y. Kojima, and L. H. Thompson (1981), '*Syakai fukushi eiwa waei yougojiten*' (Social welfare and related services glossary: English–Japanese Japanese–English), Tokyo: Seishin shobo.

Ogasawara, Yūji (1991), 'Rōjin fukushi sa-bisu to kaigo manpawa-' (Care services for the elderly and care manpower), *Zusetsu Rōnennsha hakusho,* Japan National Council of Social Welfare. pp. 122–136.

Sasaki, Takao (2005), 'Ho-muherupa- seido no rekishi oyobi kenshū no hensen—kaisei kaigo hoken seidō he no taiō wo shiya ni irete' (The history of and transition in training in the home-help system: placing responses to the revision of the Long-term Care Insurance System into our field of vision), Shukutoku daigaku shakai fukushi kenkyūjyo (The Research Institution of Social Welfare, Shukutoku University), *Sōgō fukushi kenkyū*, no.10. pp. 76–90.

Suga, Yoshiaki (2001), 'Kaigo fukushi no rekishiteki tenkai' (The historical development of care work), in Furukawa Kōjun and Satō Toyomichi (eds), *Kaigo fukushi* (Care work), Tokyo: Yūhikaku. pp. 45–62.

Takaki, Kazumi (2006, February), 'Ho-muherupusa-bisu seisaku no suii—kango kaigo rōdōsha no sabetsuteki riyou kōzō no tenkai' (Transitions in home help policy: the development of a discriminatory utilization structure for nursing and care labor), *Chingin to Shakai Hoshō*, no. 1411. pp. 4–30.

Wærness, Kari (1987), 'On the rationality of caring,' in Anne Showstack Sassoon (ed.), *Women and the State: The Shifting Boundaries of Public and Private*, London: Routledge and Hutchinson, pp. 207–34.

Wærness, Kari (2004), 'Social research, political theory and the ethics of care in a global perspective,' in Hanne Marlene Dahl and Tine Rask Eriksen (eds), *Dilemmas of Care in the Nordic Welfare State: Continuity and Change*, Ashgate. pp. 15–30.

Wærness, Kari (2008), 'Epilogue: the united voices of care workers and care researchers,' in Sirpa Wrede, Lea Henriksson, Håkon Høst, Stina Johansson and Betina Dybbroe (eds), *Care Work in Crisis: Reclaiming the Nordic Ethos of Care*, Malmö, Sweden: Studentlitteratur. pp. 363–374.

Materials and statistics

Alzheimer's' Association Japan, http://www2f.biglobe.ne.jp [July 10, 2009].

Division of Statistics, Ministry of Public Management, Home Affairs, Posts, and Telecommunications (Japan) 1972–2005, *Labour Force Research.*

Mainichi, Sankei Newspaper, July 13, 2009.

Ministry of Health, Labour, and Welfare (Japan) 2000, *Rōjin-hoken-fukushi-kyoku shinko-ka katyō tsuuchi dai 76 gō* (A notification from manager of Policy Promotion, in the Division of Health and Welfare of Elderly, No. 76).

Ministry of Health, Labour, and Welfare (Japan) 2001–2006, *Kaigo sa-bisu shisetsu jigyōsyo chōsa* (The research reports of care institutions and care providers).

Ministry of Health, Labour, and Welfare (Japan) 2002, *Ministry of Health, Labour and Welfare White Paper (Kōsei Hakusho), 2001.*

Ministry of Health, Labour, and Welfare (Japan) 2006, *Kaigo hoken seido kaikaku no gaiyō—kaigo hoken hō kaisei to kaigo hōsyū kaitei* (Outline of the LTCI reform—revision of the LTCI law and service contribution).

Ministry of Health, Labour, and Welfare (Japan) 2007, *Ministry of Health, Labour, and Welfare White Paper (Kōsei Hakusho), 2006.*

Ministry of Health, Labour, and Welfare (Japan) 2009, *Ministry of Health, Labour, and Welfare White Paper (Kōsei Hakusho), 2008.*

Population Division of the Department of Economic and Social Affairs of the United Nations Secretariat, *World Population Prospects: The 2008 Revision.*

Rengo (Japan Trade Union Confederation) 1995, *Rengo Jittai Chōsa. 55 sai ijyō no kaigō wo hitsuyō to shiteiru wo kakaeru kazoku no jittai chōsa.* (Research report of elderly care condition for family carers who care for old parents over 55 years old).

Statistiska centralbyrån (Sweden), *Sysselsättningsintensitet 1976–2004*, http://www.scb.se [February 2008].

Statistisk sentralbyrå (Norway), *Arbeidskraftundersøkelsen 2001. 1. Personer i alderen 16-74 år etter kjønn og arbeidsstyrkestatus. Årsgjennomsnitt. 1000 og prosent.* http://www.ssb.no [February 2008].

The Tenth Quality-of-life Policy Council (July 1984 – July 1986) 1986, *'Daijyuji kokumin seikatsu shingikai sōgō seisakubukai seisaku iinnkai houkoku* (The Report of the 10th Quality-of life Policy Council's total policy committee).

The Women's Association for the Better Aging Society, http://www7.ocn.ne.jp [July 10, 2009].

Chapter 4

Ainoya Yasutaka, Kunimitsu Kakiuchi, and Masaaki Ogawa (eds) (2001), *Kaigo hoken no genkai: Nihon no fukushi ronten to kadai* (Limits of the long-term care insurance: problems and issues in the Japanese welfare), Ōtsuki shoten.

Banzai, Tomohide (1999), *Jendā to ie bunka* (Gender and the *ie* culture), Shakai hyōron sha.

Campbell, John Creighton (2002), *Japanese Social Policy in Comparative Perspective*, World Bank Institute Working Papers, World Bank Institute.

Clifford, Mark E. (2003), 'The stars of Asia—entrepreneurs: Mitsuru Haruyama, Founder, Handi Network International, Japan,' *Business Week*, June 9, http://www.businessweek.com/magazine/content/03_23/b3836609.htm.

Esping-Andersen, Gøsta (1990), *The Three Worlds of Welfare Capitalism*, New Jersey: Princeton University Press.

Fraser, Nancy (1997), *Justice Interruptus: Critical Reflections on the 'Postsocialist' Condition*, London: Routledge.

Goodin, Robert (1985), *Protecting the Vulnerable: Re-Analysis of our Social Responsibilities*, Chicago University Press.

Hiraoka, Kōichi (2008), 'Kea shijōka no kanōsei to genkai' (Possibilities and limits of marketization of care), in Chizuko Ueno, Yukiko Ōkuma, Mari Ōsawa, Naohiko Jinno, and Yoshiya Fukuda (eds), *Kea sono shisō to jissen 5: Kea o sasaeru shikumi* (Theory and practice in care 5: mechanisms that support care), Iwanami shoten, pp. 125–42.

Ichihara, Akiko (2006), 'Misora intabyu: gesuto o kagayakaseru "guddo taimu kurabu" towa?' (Misora interview: what is the "good time club" that lets our guests shine?), *Misora*, vol. 2.

Ichihara, Akiko (2007, December 1), interview with the author of the present essay at Tsuru no sato.

Japan Times (2005), 'Preventive care for the elderly (editorial),' *Japan Times*, Friday, July 15.

Jinno, Masahiko (2008), 'Kea o sasaeru shikumi: bijon to sekkei' (Mechanisms supporting care: visions and planning), in Chizuko Ueno, Yukiko Ōkuma, Mari Ōsawa, Naohiko Jinno, and Yoshiya Fukuda (eds), *Kea sono shisō to jissen 5: Kea o sasaeru shikumi*, Iwanami shoten, pp. 1–26.

Kasaya, Harumi (2004), 'Fukushi rōdō no jendā kadai' (Gender-related issues in social welfare labor), in Sugimoto Kiyoe (ed.), *Feminisuto fukushi seisaku genron: Shakai fukushi no atarashii kenkyū shikaku o motomete* (Basic theories in gender and social welfare politics), Mineruva shobō, pp. 23–41.

Kasuga, Kisuyo (2001), *Kaigo mondai no shakaigaku* (Sociology of welfare problematics), Iwanami shoten.

Kasuga, Kisuyo (2003), 'Kōreisha kaigo rinri no paradaimu tenkan to kea rōdō' (The paradigm shift in the ethics of care of the elderly and the care labor), in *Shisō* 2003 (11), pp. 216–36.

Katō, Sonoko (2001), 'Shakai fukushi seisaku to fukushi rōdō' (Social welfare politics and welfare labor), in Ueda Akira, Kakiuchi Kunimitsu, and Katō Sonoko (eds), *Shakai fukushi rōdō no senmonsei to genjitsu* (Specialized nature of social welfare labour and the reality), Kyoto: Kamogawa shuppan, pp. 14–35.

Kittay, Eva Feder (1999), *Love's Labor: Essays on Women, Equality, and Dependency*, London: Routledge.

Kurube, Noriko (2008) 'Sābisu kakusa ni miru kea shisutemu no kadai,' in Chizuko Ueno, Yukiko Ōkuma, Mari Ōsawa, Naohiko Jinno, and Yoshiya Fukuda (eds), *Kea sono shisō to jissen 5: Kea o sasaeru shikumi*, Iwanami shoten, pp. 27–52.

Miyamoto, Tarō (1999), 'Fukushi tagen shugi no riron to genjitsu' (Social welfare pluralism theory and the reality), in Kawaguchi Kiyofumi and Miyazawa Kenji (eds), *Fukushi shakai to hieiri kyōdō sekutā* (Social welfare state and the non-profit sector), Nihon keizai hyōron sha, pp. 179–203.

Morimiya, Katsuko (2006), 'Kaigo bijinesu kenkyū (VI): Yūryō rōjin hōmu no shōhisha mondai' (Study on the nursing care business: private nursing homes seen from the perspective of the consumers), *Keiei ronshū, Bunkyō gakuin daigaku kiyō*, 16 (1), pp. 101–15.

Nakai, Kiyoko (2004), 'Kōreishakai to kaigo no shakaika' (Aging society and socialization of the care), in Kiyoe Sugimoto (ed.), *Feminisuto fukushi seisaku genron: Shakai fukushi no atarashii kenkyū shikaku o motomete*, Mineruva shobō, pp. 43–63.

Osako, Masako (2006), 'For-profit corporations enter the licensed private senior housing (Yūryō rōjin hōmu) sector in droves,' *From Japan Now, http://longevity.ilcjapan.org/f_issues/0701.html.*

Saito, Yayoi (2007), 'Care providers in the Long-Term Care Insurance System in Japan: the potential of and challenges faced by social enterprises' paper presented at the NTNU Japan Seminar 2007 'Eldercare in Japan and Norway: Organization and Quality', hosted by NTNU's Japan Program, 20–21 September 2007, Trondheim.

Sakamoto, Tadatsugi (ed.) (2003), *Gendai shakai fukushi no shomondai: Kaigo hoken no genjō to zaisei o chūshin ni* (Various problems in today's social welfare: focusing on the realities of the long-term care insurance and its financing), Kōyō shobō.

Sugimoto, Kiyoe (1997), *Josei ka suru fukushi shakai* (Feminization of social welfare society), Keisō shobō.

Sugimoto, Kiyoe (2004), 'Joshō: Feminisuto shakai fukushi gaku o mezashite' (Prelude: aiming at feminist social welfare) in Kiyoe Sugimoto (ed.),

Feminisuto fukushi seisaku genron: Shakai fukushi no atarashii kenkyū shikaku o motomete, Mineruva shobō, pp. 1–21.

Tsuru no sato (2008), 'Shōgai kuraseru "anshin" no kurashi: asisteddo naasingu ando rivingu Tsuru no sato' (A life-time home with secure living: assisted nursing home, Tsuro no sato). http://www.gsen.or.jp/cgi-bin/tsurunosato/top.cgi [Dec. 20, 2008]

Ueno, Chizuko (2005), *Oiru junbi: kaigo surukoto, sarerukoto* (Preparation for old age: caring and being cared for), Gakuyō shobō.

Ueno, Chizuko (2007), 'Chihō jichi, enu pî ō, josei' (Local autonomy, NPO, and women), in Mariko Adachi, Kumiko Ida, Ryōko Kimura, and Kimie Kumayasu (eds), *Feminisuto poritikusu no shintenkai: rōdō, kea, gurōbalizeishon* (A new development in feminist politics: labour, care and globalization), Akashi shoten, pp. 177–97.

Wærness, Kari (1984), 'The rationality of caring,' *Economic and Industrial Democracy*, 5, pp. 185–211.

Wærness, Kari (1999), 'Omsorg, omsorgsarbeid og omsorgsrasjonalitet: Refleksjoner over en sosialpolitisk diskurs' (Care, care work, and the rationality of care: reflections over a social political discourse), in Kirsten Thorsen and Kari Wærness (eds), *Blir omsorgen borte?: eldre omsorgens hverdag i den sen moderne velferdsstaten* (Will care disappear?: everyday reality in the care of the elderly in the late modern welfare state), Oslo: Gyldendal, pp. 46–61.

Wærness, Kari (2008) 'Epilogue,' in Sirpa Wrede, Lea Henriksson, Håkon Høst, Stina Johansson, and Betina Dybbroe (eds), *Care Work in Crisis: Reclaiming the Nordic Ethos of Care*, Malmo, Sweden: Studentlitteratur, pp. 363–74.

Yamanaka, Einosuke (2001), 'Hajimeni' (Foreword), in Einosuke Yamanaka, Eiko Takeyasu, Hiromi Sone, and Reiko Shiraishi (eds), *Kaigo to kazoku* (Care and the family), Waseda daigaku shuppan bu, pp. 1–19.

Yuki, Yasuhiro (2008), *Kaigo: genba kara no kenshō* (Care: observations from where it takes place), Iwanami shoten.

Chapter 5

Christensen, K. (2005), 'The modernisation of power in Norwegian home care services,' in H. M. Dahl and T. Rask Eriksen (eds.), *Dilemmas of Care in the Nordic Welfare State: Continuity and Change*, Aldershot: Ashgate, pp. 33–46.

Elster, E. (1995), 'Hjemmetjenestens personale: Hjemmehjelper,' in E. Elster and T. Hegerstrøm (eds.), *Kommunale hjemmetjenester—mangfold og muligheter* (Public home help services—diversity and possibilities), Oslo: Tano Aschehoug, pp. 128–37.

Gough, R. (1987), *Hemhjälp till gamla* (Home help for the elderly), Stockholm: Forskningsrapport 54, Arbetslivscentrum.

Mesle, C. R. (1983), 'Aesthetic value and relational power: an essay on personhood,' in *Process Studies*.

Næss, S. and K. Wærness (1996), *Bedre omsorg? Kommunal eldreomsorg 1980–1995* (Better care? Public care for the elderly 1980–1995), Bergen: Sefos.

Rønning, R. (2004), *Omsorg som vare? Kampen om omsorgens sjel i norske kommuner* (Care as commodity? The fight for the soul of care in Norwegian municipalities), Oslo: Gyldendal akademisk forlag.

Szebehely, M. (1995), *Vardagens organisering: om vårdbiträden och gamla i hemtjänsten* (Organizing workdays: on care and elderly within home care), Lund: Arkiv forlag.

Szebehely, M. (ed.) (2003), *Hemhjälp i Norden—illustrationer och reflektioner* (Home help in the Nordic countries—illustrations and reflections), Stockholm: Studentlitteratur.

Thorsen, K. (2003), 'Kjønn, makt og avmakt i omsorgstjenestene' (Gender, power and powerlessness within care services), in L. W. Isaksen (ed.), *Omsorgens pris* (The price of care), Oslo: Gyldendal norsk forlag, pp. 128–61.

Wæness, K. (1982), *Kvinneperspektiver på sosialpolitikken* (Female perspectives on social policy), Oslo: Universitetsforlaget.

Wæness, K. (1999), 'Omsorg, omsorgsarbeid og omsorgsrasjonalitet—refleksjoner over en sosialpolitisk diskurs,' (Care, care work and care rationality—reflections on a social political discourse), in K. Thorsen and K.Wærness (eds), *Blir omsorgen borte? Eldreomsorgens hverdag i den senmoderne velferdsstaten* (Is care being lost? Elderly care realities in the late modern welfare state), Oslo: Ad Notam Gyldendal, pp. 46–62.

Chapter 6

Kobe Research Institute of Urban Issues (Zaidanhojin Kobe toshimondai kenkyujyo) (2002), *Chiiki wo sasae kasseikasuru kommunitei bizinesu no kadai to aratana hōkōsei* (Challenges and direction of community business), Kobe: Kobe Research Institute of Urban Issues (Zaidanhojin Kobe toshimondai kenkyujyo).

Ministry of Health and Welfare (1994), *Annual Report on Health and Welfare 1992–1993*.

Ministry of Health and Welfare (1998), *Annual Report on Health and Welfare 1996–1997: For improved 'Health' and 'Quality of Life.'*

Ministry of Health and Welfare (2000), *Annual Report on Health and Welfare 1998–1999: Social Security and National Life.*

Ministry of Health, Labour, and Welfare (2007), *Overview of the Revision of the Long-term Care Insurance System: Amendment of the Long-term Care Insurance Law and Long-term Care Fee.*

Nakamura, Yuichi, Yoko Kojima, and L. H. Tomson, *Social Welfare and Related Services Glossary*, Tokyo: Seishinsyobo Press.

Nihon Iryo Seisakukiko, *Annual Report on Medical Care 1998* (*Iryō Hakusyo 1998*), Tokyo: Nihon Iryō Kikaku.

Pestoff, Victor A. (1998), *Beyond the Market and State: Social Enterprises and Civil Democracy in a Welfare Society*, Aldershot: Ashgate.

Saito, Yayoi (2005), 'Hyuman saabisu ni okeru komyuniti bijinesu no genjyō to kanousei—kaigo saabisu wo jirei toshite–' (Current state and potential of community businesses for providing human services: a case study of elderly care providers), in Nira Research Report No. 20050046, *Research Concerning Revitalizing Local Communities and Forming Broad Regional Government*, Osaka: Research Institute of Society and Economy in Kansai (Kansai syakai keizai kenkyujyo), chapter 5, section 2.

Socialstyrelsen (National Board of Health and Social Welfare) 2003, *Konkurrensutsättning och entreprenader inom äldreomsorgen: Utvecklingslaget 2003* (Competitive condition and enterprises in elderly care in Sweden 2003), Stockholm: Socialstyrelsen.

Tsutsui, Noriko (2003), *Nihon ni okeru borantea hattenn no rekishi* (History of voluntary work in Japan), Osaka Association of Volunteer (ed.), Tokyo: Chuohoki Press.

Yamanoi, Kazunori and Yayoi Saito (1994), *Taiken rupo: Nihon no kōreisya fukushi* (Elderly care in Japan), Tokyo: Iwanami Press.

Materials and statistics

Cabinet Office, Government of Japan (2009), http://www.npo-homepage.go.jp [July 30, 2009].

Chapter 7

Christensen, K. (1997), Omsorg og arbejde, En sociologisk studie af ændringer i denhjemmebaserte omsorgen (Care and work, a sociological study of change in the home based care services), Dr.polit.avhandling, Sosiologisk Institutt, Universitetet i Bergen.

Eliasson, R. (1992), 'Omsorg och rationalitet' (Care and rationality) in R. Eliasson (ed.), *Egenheter och allmänheter en antologi om omsorg och omsorgens villkor* (Peculiarity and generality in care and care condition), Lund: Studentlitteratur.

Gough, R. (1987), *Hemhjälp till gamla* (Home help for the elderly), Stockholm: Forskningsrapport 54.Arbetslivscentrum.

Liljeström, R. and Özgalda, E. (1980), *Kommunals kvinnor på livets trappa* (Female workers in the Swedish municipal workers union on the stair of life), Stockholm: Svenska kommunalarbetarförbundet.

Næss, S. and K. Wærness (1996), Bedre omsorg? Kommunal eldreomsorg 1980–1995 (Better care? Municipal elderly care services 1980–1995), Bergen: SEFOS.

Nordhus, I. H., L. W. Isaksen, and K. Wærness (1987), *De fleste gamle er kvinner* (Most of the elderly are women), Bergen: Universitetsforlaget.

Simonen, L. (1990), Contradictions of the Welfare State, Women and Caring, doctoral dissertation, University of Tampere.

Szebehely, M. (1995), *Vardagens organisering. Om vårdbiträden och gamla i hemtjänsten* (Organization of daily life: care workers and the elderly in the home help services), Lund: Arkiv Forlag.

Vabø, M. (2007), Organisering or velferd. Hjemmetjenesten i en ideologisk brytningstid (Organizing for welfare: home care services in our time of ideological upheaval), Oslo: Dr.philos- avhandling. Institutt for sosiologi og samfunnsgeografi., universitetet i Oslo.

Wærness, K. (1978), *Hjemnehjelperne-den modeme velferdsstats hushjelper* (Home helpers—the modern welfare state's house maids), Tidsskrift for samfunnsforskning, vol. 19.

Wærness, K. (1984), 'The rationality of caring,' *Economic and Industrial Democracy*, 5, pp. 185–211.

Wærness, K. (1995), 'En offentlig tjeneste i spenningsfeltet mellom ulike kulturer' in S. Johansson (ed.), *Sjukhus och hem som arbetsplass* (Hospital and home as a working place), Stockholm/Oslo: Bonniers/ Unlversitetsforlaget.

Wrede, Scupa, Hea Henrelesson, Hahon Host, Stiva Johansson, and Betina Dybroe (eds) (2008), *Care Work in Crisis: Reclaiming the Nordic Ethos of Care,* Stockholm: Studentlittertur.

Chapter 8

Andersen, Jørgen Goul (2006), 'Reforming the Danish welfare state: new public management, user influence, and citizens' rights,' International Workshop on Public Service Reform in Scandinavian Welfare States: Towards More Inclusive Societies, March 9, Tokyo.

Asahi Shimbun (Asahi newsletter) (2006), 15 October.

Avery, Gayle C. (2005), *Leadership for Sustainable Futures: Achieving Success in a Competitive World*, Cheltenham: Edward Elgar.

Belinszki, Eszter, Katrin Hansen, and Ursula Müller (Hg.) (2003), *Diversity Management*, Münster: LIT Verlag.

Blinder, Alan (2006), 'Offshoring: the next industrial revolution?', *Foreign Affairs*, March/April, pp. 113–28.

Blmqvist, Paula (2006), 'NPM and Swedish welfare services: the impact of new ideas', International Workshop on Public Service Reform in Scandinavian Welfare States: Towards More Inclusive Societies, March 9, Tokyo.

Ciulla, Joanne B. (ed.) (1998), *Ethics, The Heart of Leadership*, Quorum Books.

Drucker, Peter Ferdinand (trans. Atsuo Ueda) (2000), *Chenji rihda no johken: Mizukara henka wo tsukuridase!* (The change lead: one can only be ahead of it!), Tokyo: Daiamondosha.

Fujiwara, Yasunobu (2007), *Seijitetsugaku no fukken* (Recovery of political philosophy), Tokyo: Shinhyoron.

Konopaske, Robert and John M. Ivancevich (2004), *Global Management and Organizational Behavior*, New York: McGraw-Hill.

Miyazawa, Kenichi (2006), 'Iryo—kaigo no fukushiteki/zaiseiteki/sangyoteki sanchoryu to sono kohsaku (Healthcare: trend for nursing care and its mixture in welfare, finance and industry),' *Iryokeizai Kenkyu,* 18 (12), pp. 79–92.

Morioka, Koji (2006), 'Misekake no jitan no kage de susumu hatarakisugi (Excess work: reality under reduced working hours),' *LRL: Labor Research Library*, 14 (12), pp. 3–6.

Plummer, Deborah L. (ed.) 2003, *Handbook of Diversity Management*, University Press of America.

Rengoh sohgo seikatsukaihatsu kenkyujo (2007), *Kurashi to syakai ni tsuiteno anketochosa* (Questionnaire survey and report on life and society), January.

Shigeru, Suzato, Kitazawa Hiroshi, and Sakurai Hitoshi (1996), *Lifusutairu To Syakaikohzo* (Lifestyle and social structure), Tokyo: Nihon Hyoronsya.

Sison, Alejo Jose G. (2003), *The Moral Capital of Leaders*, Cheltenham: Edward Elgar, *Dagens Nyheter* 2007-04-15.

Yamada, Masahiro (2006), *Shinbyohdohsyakai: kibohkakusa wo koete* (New equal society: beyond expectation gap society), Tokyo: Bungeisyunju.

Yoisyakai wo tsukuru kohkyosahbisu wo kangaerukenkyukai (2006), 'Kenkyukaihohkoku: yoisyakai no kohkyosahbisu wo kangaeru: zaiseisaikensyugi wo koe yuhkoh ni kinohsuru hodoyoiseihu wo (Research report: consider public service for better society: Effective and balanced government over financial reconstruction)'.

Appendix

Table A: Population, fertility rate and life expectancy (2006)

	Japan	Norway	Sweden	Denmark	Finland
Population (people)	127,769,510	4,660,673	9,080,506	5,434,567	5,266,266
Ratio of population aged 65 and over (%)	20.82	14.68	17.33	15.26	16.23
Fertility rate[1]	1.32	1.90	1.85	1.85	1.84
Life expectancy[2] (total)	82.4	80.6	80.8	78.4	79.5
Life expectancy[2] (men)	79.0	78.2	78.7	76.1	75.9
Life expectancy[2] (women)	85.8	82.9	82.9	80.7	83.1

Notes: 1) Number of children born to women aged 15 to 49. Life expectancy: Number of years.

Source: OECD. OECD Factbook 2009: Economic, Environmental and Social Statistics. Statistical profiles 2009, Stat Extracts (http://stats.oecd.org [January 20, 2010])

Table B: GDP per capita, employment and unemployment rate (2007)

	Japan	Norway	Sweden	Denmark	Finland
GDP per capita[1]	33626.15	53476.60	36603.11	35961.42	34717.98
Real GDP growth[2]	2.1	3.1	2.5	1.6	4.5
Employment rate[3] (total)	70.68	77.55	75.65	77.33	70.46
Employment rate[3] (men)	81.72	80.38	78.02	81.28	72.38
Employment rate[3] (women)	59.48	74.63	73.21	73.30	68.49
Unemployment rate[4] (total)	3.9	2.6	6.2	3.8	6.9
Unemployment rate[4] (men)	3.9	2.6	5.9	3.4	6.5
Unemployment rate[4] (women)	3.7	2.5	6.4	4.1	7.2

Notes: 1) Gross Domestic Product, US dollars, current prices and PPPs. 2) Annual growth of Gross Domestic Product in percentage. 3) Share of persons of working age (15 to 64 years) in employment. 4) Unemployment person as a percentage of civilian labor force.

Source: OECD. OECD Factbook 2009: Economic, Environmental and Social Statistics. Statistical profiles 2009, Stat Extracts (http://stats.oecd.org [January 20, 2010])

Table C: Social expenditure, tax revenue (2005)

(as a percentage of GDP)

	Japan	Norway	Sweden	Denmark	Finland
Public expenditure on health	6.7	7.6	7.5	7.9	6.2
Public social expenditure	18.6	21.6	29.4	26.9	26.1
Total tax revenue	27.36	43.52	49.48	50.73	43.93

Source: OECD. OECD Factbook 2009: Economic, Environmental and Social Statistics. Statistical profiles 2009, Stat Extracts (http://stats.oecd.org [January 20, 2010])

Table D: Income inequality: Gini coefficient level (2006)

	Japan	Norway	Sweden	Denmark	Finland
Gini coefficient level	0.32	0.28	0.23	0.23	0.27
Gini coefficient rank in the OECD 30 countries	20	11	2	1	7

Source: OECD. OECD Factbook 2009: Economic, Environmental and Social Statistics. Statistical profiles 2009, Stat Extracts (http://stats.oecd.org [January 20, 2010])

Table E: Trends in the population aging rate (Norway, Sweden and Japan)

	1950	1955	1960	1965	1970	1975	1980	1985	1990	1995	2000	2005
Japan	4.9 (0.4)	5.3 (0.6)	5.7 (0.7)	6.2 (0.8)	7.0 (0.9)	7.9 (1.1)	9.1 (1.4)	10.2 (1.8)	12.0 (2.4)	14.4 (3.1)	17.2 (3.8)	19.9 (4.9)
Norway	9.7 (1.7)	10.2 (1.8)	11.1 (1.9)	12.0 (2.0)	12.9 (2.2)	13.7 (2.5)	14.8 (3.0)	15.7 (3.4)	16.3 (3.7)	15.9 (4.0)	15.0 (4.3)	14.5 (4.6)
Sweden	10.3 (1.5)	10.9 (1.6)	12.0 (1.9)	12.7 (2.1)	13.7 (2.3)	15.1 (2.7)	16.3 (3.2)	17.9 (4.0)	17.8 (4.3)	17.5 (4.7)	17.2 (5.0)	17.2 (5.4)

Note: The rate in parenthesis represents the percentage of the population aged 80 and over.

Source: Based on Population Division of the Department of Economic and Social Affairs of the United Nations Secretariat. *World Population Prospects: The 2008 Revision.*

Table F: Changes in the number of primary insured person(Japan)

(people)

2000	2001	2002	2003	2004	2005	2006	2007
21,654,769	22,473,297	23,223,722	23,981,379	24,528,385	25,160,699	25,935,454	26,822,941

as of the end of April in each year

Source: Ministry of Health, Labour and Welfare (Japan). *Annual Health, Labour and Welfare Report 2007–2008.* Ref-pp. 229

Table G: Changes in the number of home help service users (Japan)

(people)

	2000	2001	2002	2003	2004	2005	2006	2007
Home help service	446,679	600,313	728,974	899,167	972,266	1,090,112	882,556	738,793
Care prevention home help service*	–	–	–	–	–	–	159,791	306,458

as of the end of September in each year

Source: Based on Ministry of Health, Labour and Welfare (Japan) 2000–2007, *Kaigo sa-bisu shisetsu jigyōsyo chosa* (The research reports of care providers).

Editor's notes: Care prevention home help service (Kaigo yobō houmon kaigo) was introduced at the time of revision of the Long-Term Care Insurance Law (enforced on April 1, 2006). According to the Law, this service is prepared for the elderly who are certificated as on the support level 1 or 2 has the contents, period and method suited for those in a slight condition to meet the purpose of "keeping and improving the life functions and preventing people from getting into the care need condition."

Table H: Changes in the number of facility services users (Japan)

(people)

	2000	2001	2002	2003	2004	2005	2006	2007
Facility Services	144,874	200,177	212,586	214,033	227,927	234,326	198,493	205,154
Other dwellings*	5,450	12,486	23,888	43,519	70,161	94,907	118,023	129,175

as of the end of September in each year

Source: Based on Ministry of Health, Labour and Welfare. *Annual Health, Labour and Welfare Report 2007–2008*. Ref-pp.229, and Ministry of Health, Labour and Welfare (Japan) 2000–2007, *Kaigo sa-bisu shisetsu jigyōsyo chosa* (The research reports of care providers).

Editors's notes: Other dwellings included 'daily-life group care for the elderly with dementia (Ninchisyō taiougata kyōdōseikatsukaigo)', 'community-oriented daily-life care service in specified facilities (chiiki mittyakugata tokutei shisetsu nyūsyosya seikatsukaigo)', and 'daily-life care service in welfare facilities for the elderly requiring care (chiiki mittyakugata kaigo rōjin fukushi nyūsyosya seikatsukaigo'. These dwellings are categorized as In-home services (Kyotaku sa-bisu) and Community-oriented services (chiiki mittyakugata sa-bisu). Users of daily-life care service in specified facilities (Tokutei shisetsu nyūsyosya seikatukaigo) are not included in the statistics for lack of data.

Table I: Financial trend of the Long-Term Care Insurance (Japan)

(Million Euro)

2000	2001	2002	2003	2004	2005	2006	2007	2008	2009
27,870	35,611	40,256	44,127	47,998	49,546	49,546	53,417*	55,740*	59,610*

Source: Based on Ministry of Health, Labour and Welfare. *Annual Health, Labour and Welfare Report 2007–2008*. Ref-pp.229.

Note: Statistics of 2000–2006 mean actual cost (Long-Term Care benefit and 10% copayment by user). Statistics of 2007–2009 mean budget.

Table J: Users of home based services, by kind of service, 1992–2008 (Norway)

(people)

	1992	1993	1994	1995	1996	1997	1998	1999
Total	**146,272**	**142,623**	**142,354**	**145,249**	**144,765**	**149,026**	**152,796**	**157,396**
Both home helpand home nursing	50,110	48,656	47,156	45,228	48,164	51,143	54,643	57,521
Home nursing only	25,316	24,538	21,964	19,982	22,479	23,858	27,068	33,211
Home help only	70,846	69,429	73,147	68,784	73,411	72,653	68,649	64,944
Unspecified users	0	0	87	11,255	711	1,372	2,436	1,720

	2000	2001	2002	2003	2004	2005	2006	2007	2008
Total	**159,669**	**161,169**	**162,112**	**161,094**	**163,415**	**164,623**	**171,226**	**161,817**	**167,442**
Both home helpand home nursing	59,229	59,095	58,789	59,896	60,460	62,119	66,558	57,490	58,971
Home nursing only	37,647	40,327	44,399	46,529	51,348	54,491	56,547	58,439	62,529
Home help only	62,793	61,747	58,924	54,669	51,607	48,013	48,121	45,888	45,942
Unspecified users	0	0	0	0	0	0	0	0	0

Notes: 10,720 persons receiving "other services" and 535 users of home nursery and/or home help were not specified, and are as from 2003 included in the total. Break in time-series. Until 2007 the number of man-years was collected by use of summary questionnaires. From 2007 the figures are collected from the IPLOS-register. Figures from 2007 and later are thus not directly comparable with figures from preceding years.

Source: Statistisk sentralbyrå (Norway). *Nursing and social care services*. (http://www.ssb.no [January 20,2010])

Table K: Residents in institutions for the elderly and disabled, 1992–2008 (Norway)

(people)

	1992	1993	1994	1995	1996	1997	1998	1999	2000	2001	2002	2003	2004	2005	2006	2007*	2008*
Total	**45,571**	**44,878**	**43,447**	**42,532**	**43,075**	**42,921**	**42,406**	**42,691**	**42,236**	**41,894**	**41,635**	**41,013**	**40,985**	**40,719**	**40,537**	**42,293**	**42,129**
Under 67 years	1,804	1,663	1,611	1,589	1,576	1,586	1,519	1,575	1,598	1,619	1,714	1,799	1,866	1,862	1,924	4,116	4,109
67–79 years	10,579	10,648	10,243	10,085	9,789	9,765	9,425	9,455	9,090	8,749	8,499	8,184	8,134	7,639	7,478	7,000	6,882
80–89 years	22,807	22,453	21,838	21,198	21,266	21,447	21,332	21,640	21,470	21,263	21,314	20,999	20,960	20,656	20,368	19,422	19,240
90 years and over	10,381	10,114	9,755	9,660	9,794	9,644	9,863	10,021	10,007	10,263	10,108	10,031	10,025	10,562	10,767	11,754	11,898
Unspecified age	0	0	0	0	650	479	267	0	71	0	0	0	0	0	0	:	0

Notes: * Break in time-series. Until 2007 the number of man-years was collected by use of summary questionnaires. From 2007 the figures are collected from the IPLOS-register. Figures from 2007 and later are thus not directly comparable with figures from preceding years.

Source: Statistisk sentralbyrå (Norway). *Nursing and social care services.* (http://www.ssb.no [January 20, 2010])

Table L: Residents in dwellings for the elderly and disabled, 1992–2008 (Norway)

(people)

	1994	1995[1]	1996[2]	1997[3]	1998[4]	1999[5]
Total	**30,260**	**32,338**	**35,254**	**38,140**	**40,617**	**43,983**
Under 67 years	9,013	9,169	9,592	10,783	11,573	12,545
67–79 years	8,437	8,647	10,053	11,133	11,275	12,293
80–89 years	10,042	10,047	11,597	13,018	13,711	14,695
90 years and over	2,070	2,121	2,523	2,912	3,260	3,564
Unspecified age	698	2,354	1,489	294	798	0

2000	2001	2002	2003	2004[1]	2005	2006	2007*	2008*
45,515	**46,023**	**46,414**	**48,087**	**47,569**	**48,821**	**50,194**	**49,288**	**51,462**
13,452	14,079	14,378	15,401	15,594	16,651	17,575	18,052	19,688
12,472	11,984	11,501	11,126	10,676	10,019	9,820	8,262	8,191
15,680	15,783	16,010	16,614	16,408	16,787	17,124	16,327	16,442
3,911	4,177	4,525	4,946	4,891	5,364	5,675	6,647	7,141
71	0	0	0	0	0	0	0	0

Notes: 1) The number of dwellings and residents are underestimated. 2) The total number of residents is not specified for 3,008 dwellings. 3)The total number of residents is not specified for 1,971 dwellings. 4) The total number of residents is not specified for 1,576 dwellings. 5) The total number of residents is not specified for 496 dwellings. * Break in time-series. Until 2007 the number of residents was collected by use of summary questionnaires. From 2007 the figures are collected from the IPLOS-register. Figures from 2007 and later are thus not directly comparable with figures from preceding years. Includes number of residents from 2006 when municipality have not been able to deliver IPLOS-data.

Source: Statistisk sentralbyrå (Norway). *Nursing and social care services.* (http://www.ssb.no [January 20, 2010])

Figure A: Structure of Long-Term Care Insurance System

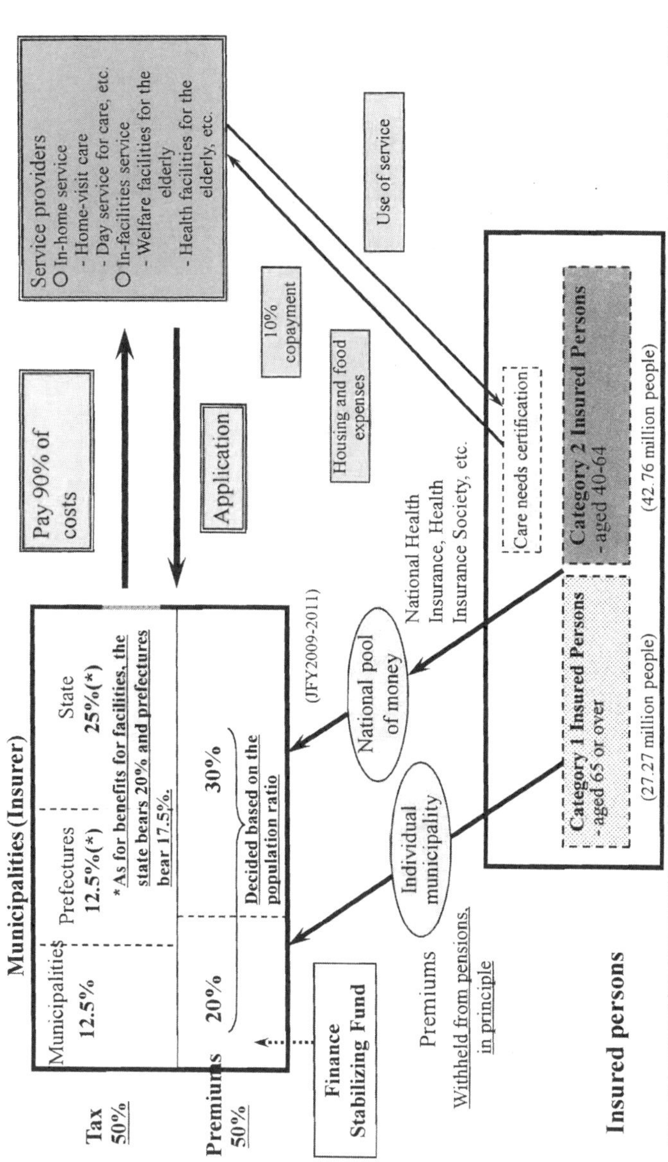

Note: The number of Category 1 insured persons is from Report on Long-Term Care Insurance Operation (provisional) (December, 2007), Ministry of Health, Labour and Welfare. The number of Category 2 insured persons is a monthly average for JFY2005, calculated from medical insurers' reports used by the Social Insurance Medical Fee Payment Fund in order to determine the amount of long-term care expenses.

Figure B: Procedures for the Use of Service

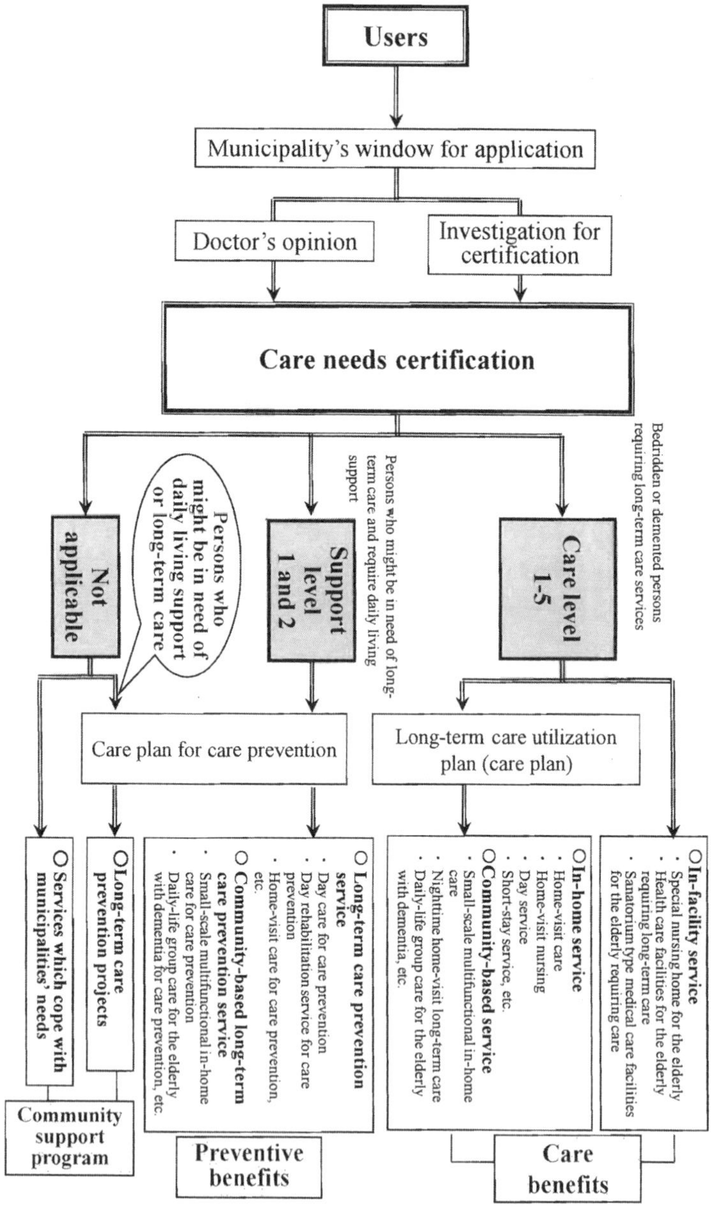

Index